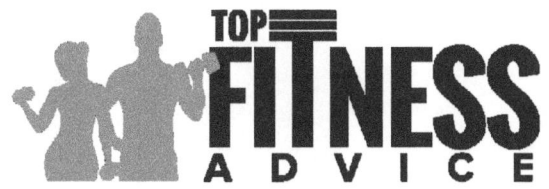

KETOGENIC COOKBOOK

67 Ketosis Recipes That Trigger Your Body Into Burning Fat As Energy All Day Long (Includes Breakfast, Lunch, Dinner)

Bruce Harlow

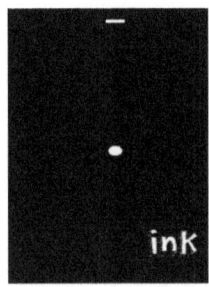

First published in 2017 by Venture Ink Publishing

Copyright © Top Fitness Advice 2019

All rights reserved.

No part of this book may be reproduced in any form without permission in writing from the author. No part of this publication may be reproduced or transmitted in any form or by any means, mechanic, electronic, photocopying, recording, by any storage or retrieval system, or transmitted by email without the permission in writing from the author and publisher.

Requests to the publisher for permission should be addressed to publishing@ventureink.co

For more information about the contents of this book or questions to the author, please contact Bruce Harlow at bruce@topfitnessadvice.com

Disclaimer

This book provides wellness management information in an informative and educational manner only, with information that is general in nature and that is not specific to you, the reader. The contents of this book are intended to assist you and other readers in your personal wellness efforts. Consult your physician regarding the applicability of any information provided in this book to you.

Nothing in this book should be construed as personal advice or diagnosis, and must not be used in this manner. The information provided about conditions is general in nature. This information does not cover all possible uses, actions, precautions, side-effects, or interactions of medicines, or medical procedures. The information in this book should not be considered as complete and does not cover all diseases, ailments, physical conditions, or their treatment.

You should consult with your physician before beginning any exercise, weight loss, or health care program. This book should not be used in place of a call or visit to a competent health-care professional. You should consult a health care professional before adopting any of the suggestions in this book or before drawing inferences from it.

Any decision regarding treatment and medication for your condition should be made with the advice and consultation of a qualified health care professional. If you have, or suspect you have, a health-care problem, then you should immediately contact a qualified health care professional for treatment.

No Warranties: The author and publisher don't guarantee or warrant the quality, accuracy, completeness, timeliness, appropriateness or suitability of the information in this book, or of any product or services referenced in this book.

The information in this book is provided on an "as is" basis and the author and publisher make no representations or warranties of any kind with respect to this information. This book may contain inaccuracies, typographical errors, or other errors.

Liability Disclaimer: The publisher, author, and other parties involved in the creation, production, provision of information, or delivery of this book specifically disclaim any responsibility, and shall not be held liable for any damages, claims, injuries, losses, liabilities, costs, or obligations including any direct, indirect, special, incidental, or consequences damages (collectively known as "Damages") whatsoever and howsoever caused, arising out of, or in connection with the use or misuse of the site and the information contained within it, whether such Damages arise in contract, tort, negligence, equity, statute law, or by way of other legal theory.

Table of Contents

Disclaimer	3
Introduction	7
How to Use This Book	11
Chapter 1: Breakfast	13
Chapter 2: Lunch	39
Chapter 3: Dinner	81
Chapter 4: Snacks	125
Conclusion	139
Final Words	141

Would you prefer to listen to my book, rather than read it?

Download the audiobook version for free!

If you go to the special link below and sign up to Audible as a new customer, you can get the audiobook version of my book completely free.

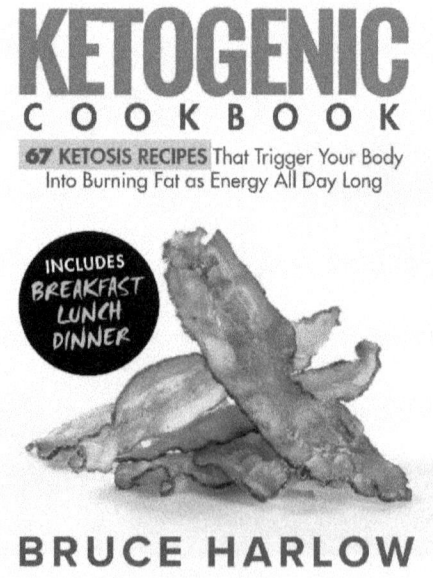

Go here to get your audiobook version for free:

TopFitnessAdvice.com/go/KetogenicCB

Introduction

When it comes to commonly held beliefs, most people have been told that eating too much fat is what makes us sick. Whilst it is true that eating too many calories in a day is bound to lead to weight gain, cutting out fat is also not the answer.

Fat came under fire because it is very calorie dense. It seems to make sense – cut out the more nutrient dense food in order to drop the number of calories that you consume.

However, if you consider that we evolved as hunter-gatherers who might have had to go without food for a day at a time or more, the picture becomes more complicated. Our bodies are not built for having such ready access to food in general and carbs in particular. Our ancestors had to go out and hunt for their food. Today though, we just stop in at the store.

Pair that with our increasingly sedentary lifestyles and it is hardly surprising that we are becoming more obese and that dieting is such a huge trend.

But, despite the fact that the typical low-fat diet has been punted as the best option for the last few decades, we are getting more obese. Despite us cutting out so much fat, we are increasingly unable to lose the weight.

But look for a minute at what it is that we do eat. We take the fat out of food and it no longer tastes so good so we add in tons of sugar. The typical Western diet consists of a high level of processed foods that are high in sugar.

However, these highly processed carbs have very little nutrient value and, because they are so processed, they have a massive impact on our blood sugar levels.

We eat the carbs and our blood sugar levels skyrocket. The body responds by increasing the production of insulin. The sugar is mopped up and your energy levels plummet again. You then crave even more carbs to fuel your body.

You quickly get caught in a vicious cycle – you need the carbs for energy but they cause your blood sugar levels to crash fairly quickly. And, after the crash, your body requires more energy and so you have to eat again.

If this happens over and over again, your body becomes less responsive to the insulin produced by it. You end up needing more insulin to clear out the excess blood sugar. More insulin is produced but it is less effective than before.

More of the glucose that is produced is left over in the blood stream and is converted to fat that gets stored in the body.

The way to get out of this cycle, is to fuel your body in a completely different way. That is where a ketogenic diet comes in to play.

Ketosis can reverse this by forcing your body to use the fat stores for energy.

The ketogenic diet turns our commonly held belief about weight-loss on its head. Instead of cutting out as much fat as possible, you eat a diet that is high in protein and that has moderate amounts of fat and that restricts carbs as much as possible.

With the lack of glucose as a fuel source in the diet, the body has no choice but to start burning through the fat stored in it. Your body actually changes its preferred fuel source over to fat – and that is why you need to increase the amount of fat that you eat.

The benefits of a ketogenic diet is that you will not feel hungry or deprived in any way and you will be able to lose weight easily. Once the initial adjustment period is over, you will find that you have a lot more energy and a greater ability to focus.

We are not going to go into the actual diet in full in this book but we do provide you with recipes that are all keto-friendly.

Good luck!

How to Use This Book

Choose one breakfast, one lunch, one dinner and either one or two snacks a day and you will start to feel the benefits for yourself.

Unless otherwise stated, the following will apply to all recipes:

- All temperatures are in Fahrenheit.

- Do no use foods that are sweetened already – if necessary, the recipe will list what sweetener to use.

- Use organic, naturally produced food wherever possible.

I hope that you are enjoying this book so far, and if you could spare 30 seconds, I would greatly appreciate you leaving a review on Amazon.com.

Chapter 1

Breakfast

1. Avocado and Salmon Egg Spread

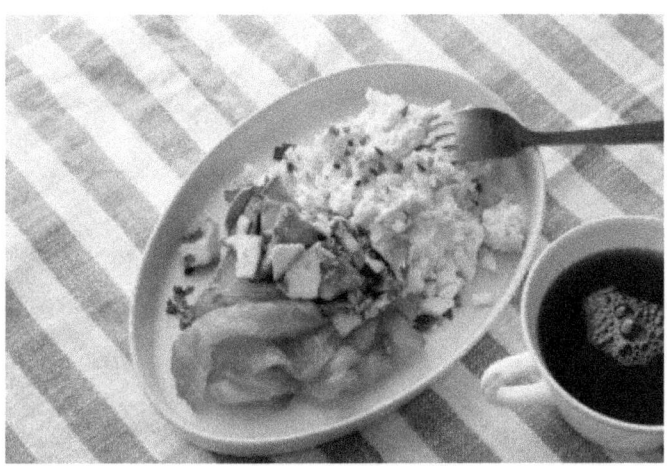

Serves 2

Ingredients

- Seasoning to taste
- 4 eggs
- 2 avocados
- 5 ounces of farm butter, take out of the refrigerator at least two hours before making the recipe
- 2 tablespoons olive oil
- 4 ounces of smoked salmon
- 1 tablespoon freshly picked parsley, very chopped up nice and finely

Method

Once again, hard boil the eggs and peel once cool to the touch. Slice the eggs nice and fine and cream them with the butter and the seasoning. Take the pit out of the avocados, peel and slice them. Top with the egg spread and some salmon and drizzle with a little olive oil.

2. Luxurious Scrambled Eggs

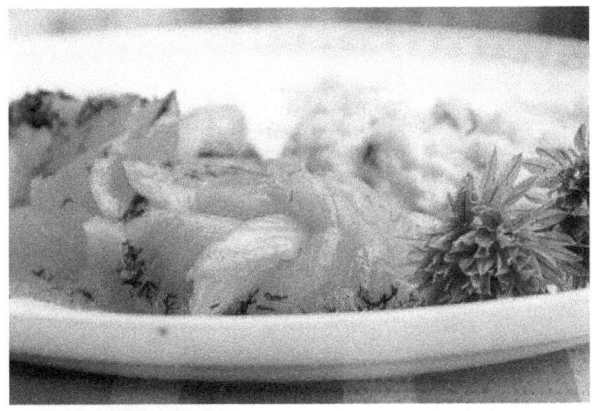

Serves 1

Ingredients

- 2 tablespoons farm butter
- 2 eggs
- 3 1/3 tablespoons double cream
- 1 – 3 slices of cured salmon
- 1 tablespoon chives, snipped into small bits
- Seasoning to taste

Method

Whisk up the eggs until frothy. Set your stove to Medium and put the farm butter into a pan. When it has melted, put the eggs in and reduce the heat to Low. Stir in the cream and let the mixture cook slowly until the eggs are done. Add in the seasoning and the chives. Serve with the salmon on the top.

3. Ham Omelet

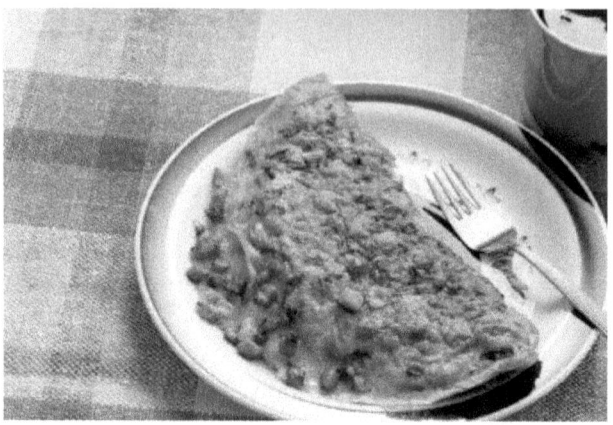

Serves 2

Ingredients

- 2 tablespoons sour cream or double cream
- 6 eggs
- Seasoning to taste
- 2 ounces of farm butter
- 3½ ounces cheese, grated
- ½ mild onion, chopped up nice and fine
- 4¾ ounces of ham, chopped up nice and fine
- ½ bell pepper of your choice, chopped up nice and fine

Method

Briskly whisk the cream and eggs until they are completely fluffy. Put in half the amount of cheese and stir again. Set your stove on Medium and let the butter melt in a heavy-bottomed frying pan. When the butter has melted, add in the onion and pepper and fry for a couple of minutes. Add the ham and fry for another minute. Pour in the egg mixture and fry until the egg starts to firm. Turn the heat down to Low and put the remaining cheese on top. Fold the omelet and serve.

4. Keto Sandwich

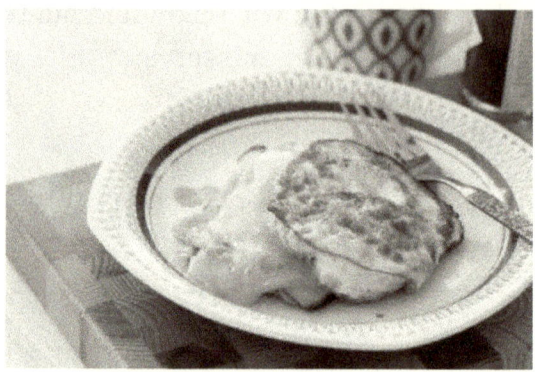

Serves 2

Ingredients

- 2 tablespoons farm butter
- 4 eggs
- A little Worcestershire sauce (Or, if you like a bit of a burn, Tabasco sauce.)
- 1 ounce of ham
- Seasoning to taste
- 2 ounces of sharp Cheddar or cheese of your choice, sliced thickly

Method

Set your stove to Medium and fry your eggs until done to your liking. Season as you like. Use one egg as a base for your sandwich. Top with the ham or whatever cold cut you like. Sprinkle cheese on top and then finish off your sandwich with a second egg. Finish it off with the sauce of your choice.

5. Breakfast Tapas

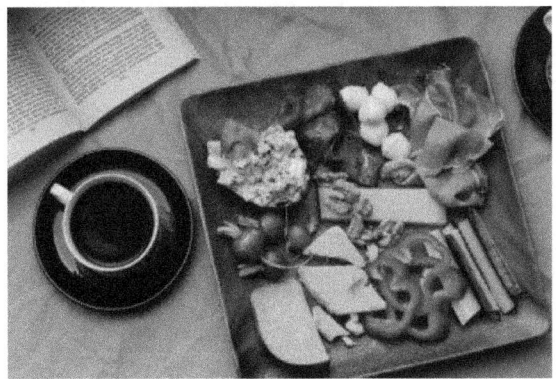

Make as Many or Few as You Like

Ingredients

- Cold cuts of your choosing like salami, prosciutto, or ham
- Cheeses of your choosing, like Cheddar, Parmesan or Mozzarella
- Freshly picked basil
- Fresh cucumber, pickles, cherry tomatoes, radishes, or peppers
- Nuts of your choosing like almonds, pecans or walnuts
- Avocadoes
- Seasoning to taste
- Mayo

Method

Take the pits out of the avocadoes, peel them and scoop out the flesh. (Reserve the shells.) Mix with enough mayo to make it creamy and season to taste. If you want a tarter flavor, you can add some lemon juice. Spoon back into the avocado shells. Slice up the cheeses, veggies and cold cuts and use them as toppings for the avocados.

6. Smoked Salmon Sandwiches

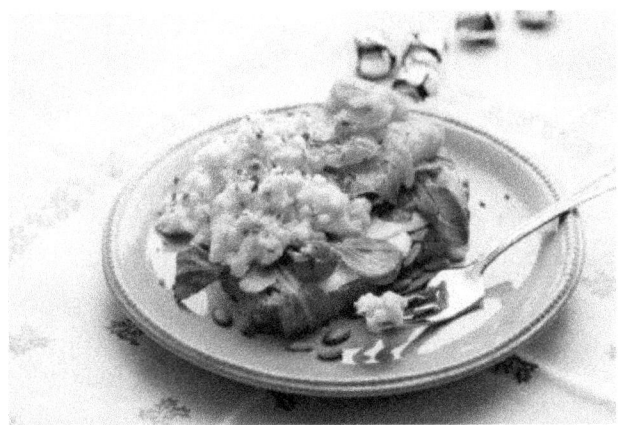

Serves 1

Ingredients for Sandwich

- 2 tablespoons double cream
- 4 eggs
- Seasoning to taste
- A dash of chili flakes
- 2 ounces of farm butter
- 2 slices of pumpkin loaf
- 2 tablespoons farm butter
- 1 ounce of lettuce
- 1 tablespoon chives, snipped into small bits
- 3¼ ounces of smoked salmon

Ingredients for Pumpkin Loaf

- 1 tablespoon baking powder
- 2 tablespoons pumpkin pie spice

- 1 teaspoon table salt
- 8 tablespoons flax seeds
- 2 tablespoons powdered psyllium husks
- 1¼ cups almond flour
- 5 ⅓ tablespoons chopped walnuts
- 1¼ cups coconut flour
- 5 ⅓ tablespoons pumpkin seeds and extra for topping
- 8 tablespoons natural apple sauce
- 3 eggs
- 4 tablespoons coconut oil
- 1 tablespoon farm butter
- 1 can pumpkin puree
- Seasoning to taste.

Method

Whisk the cream and the eggs together until frothy. Set your stove to Med-High and put the butter into a heavy-based frying pan. Put the eggs mix in and scramble. Season to taste. (If you are using the chili flakes, this is where to add them.)

Toast a couple of slices of bread – choose to make your own, according to the recipe here, or use bread that is low-carb. Butter the slices of toast. Put some lettuce on the bread and top with the eggs. Finish off with the chives and the salmon.

Pumpkin Loaf: Set your oven to 400. Oil a standard bread tin with the butter. Mix the dry ingredients together well. In a separate bowl, mix the remaining ingredients together and then blend into the dry mix. Mux until you get a smooth batter.

Place in the baking tin and top with pumpkin seeds if you like. Put on one of the low racks in your oven. Bake for about 60 minutes or so. Check for doneness by inserting a skewer. (If the skewer comes out clean, the bread is done.)

7. Halloumi Scramble

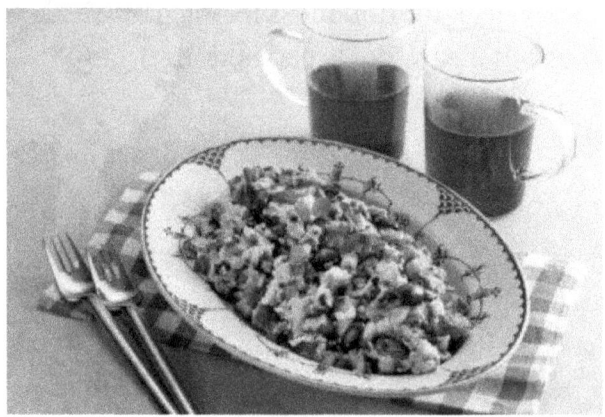

Serves 2

Ingredients

- 4½ ounces of bacon, sliced into cubes
- 5 – 6 eggs
- 3½ ounces of halloumi cheese, sliced into cube
- 8 tablespoons freshly picked parsley, chopped up nice and finely up
- 2 scallions, chopped up nice and finely up
- 8 tablespoons olives, pits removed and chopped up nice and finely up
- Seasoning to taste
- 2 tablespoons olive oil

Method

Set your stove to Med-High and warm up the oil in a heavy-based frying pan. Add the scallions, halloumi and bacon and fry until it starts to turn golden and the bacon is crisp. Whisk the eggs, season as you like and add the parsley. Add it to your frying pan and scramble. Reduce the heat to Low, stir in the olives and cook until the eggs are done to your liking.

8. Early Morning Fritters

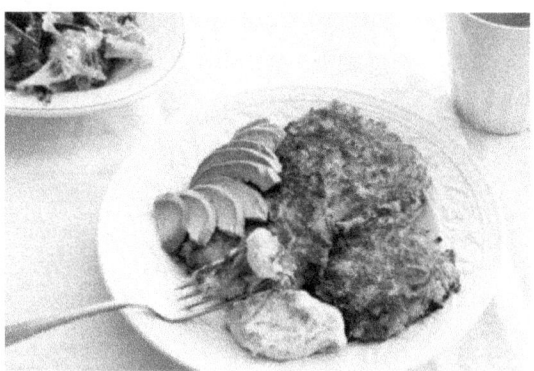

Serves 1

Ingredients

- ½ pound halloumi cheese
- 1 pound rutabaga
- 4 eggs
- 1 teaspoon turmeric
- 3 tablespoons coconut flour
- 1 teaspoon table salt
- 4 ounces of farm butter to fry the patties in
- 1 tablespoon ranch seasoning
- ¼ teaspoon pepper
- 1 cup mayo
- Ranch Dressing

Method

Clean the rutabaga well and peel it. Either process or grate it until fine. Grate the cheese as well. Mix all of the ingredients, except the butter, well and let them marinate for a little bit. Divide the mixture up into twelve evenly sized balls and flatten to form patties. Set your stove to Med-High. Place the butter into a frying pan and melt. Add the patties and fry until golden brown on both sides.

9. Cheese and Mushroom Frittata

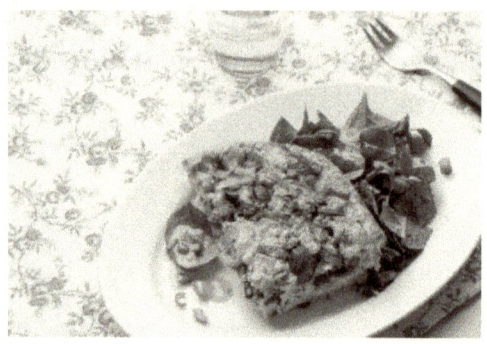

Serves 4

Ingredients for Frittata

- 3¼ ounces of farm butter
- 1 pound mushrooms
- 6 scallions, chopped up nice and fine
- 1 teaspoon table salt
- 1 tablespoon freshly picked parsley
- ½ teaspoon powdered black pepper
- 4 ounces of leafy greens
- ½ pound cheese, grated
- 10 eggs
- 1 cup mayo

Ingredients for Vinaigrette

- 1 tablespoon white wine vinegar
- 4 tablespoons olive oil
- Seasoning to taste

Method

Set your oven at 350. Mix the ingredients for the vinaigrette well and put to one side. Slice up the mushrooms. How big you make the chunks depends on your personal preference.

Set your stove to Med-High and put two-thirds of the butter in a pan. When it has melted, fry the mushrooms until they are softened and reduce the heat to Medium.

Grease an oven-proof dish with the remaining butter. Mix the mushrooms and the scallion and add seasoning as you like. Stir in the parsley. Mix together the mayo, cheese and eggs in a clean bowl. Season as required. Put the scallion/ mushroom mix into the oven-proof container and then pour over the egg mixture.

Bake until it starts to turn brown and is cooked through. It will take around half an hour or so. Allow to cool a little before serving and then serve on a bed of leafy greens and topped with your vinaigrette.

10. Egg Muffins

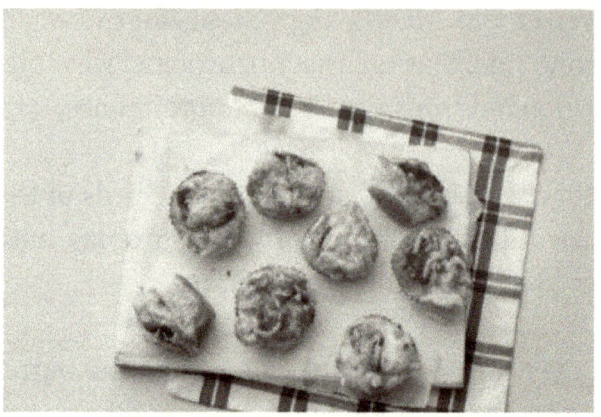

Serves 2

Ingredients

- 1 – 2 scallions, chopped up nice and fine
- 6 eggs
- 4 – 8 wafer thin slices of bacon or salami
- 1 tablespoon pesto of your choice (You can leave it out if you want)
- 3½ ounces of cheese, grated
- Seasoning to taste

Method

Set your oven at 350. Chop up the meat nice and fine. Mix together the pesto, if using, and eggs. Season to taste. Stir in the cheese. Grease a muffin tin and fill each well up to half-way. Sprinkle the meat over the top. Bake until the muffins are done – it should take about 15 minutes or so.

11. Herby, Buttery Eggs

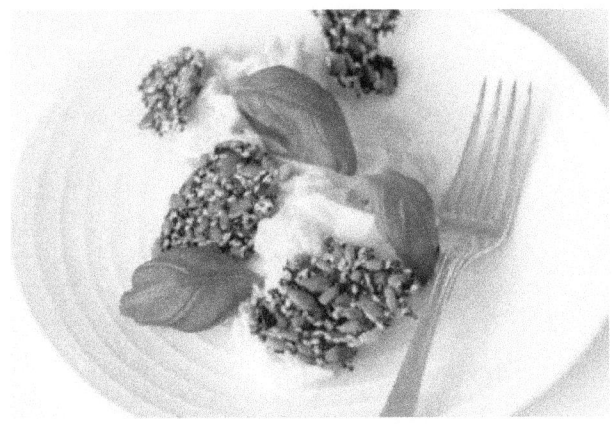

Serves 1

Ingredients

- 2 tablespoons coconut cream or sour cream
- 2 eggs
- Salt
- Grated cheese to taste
- Farm butter

Method

Set the stove to Low and heat up the butter in a frying pan. In the meantime, mix the eggs, cream and seasoning to taste. When the butter has melted, scramble the eggs until done to your liking. Melt farm butter in a pan on low heat. Mix together eggs and liquid, salt and add to the pan.

12. Low-Carb Porridge

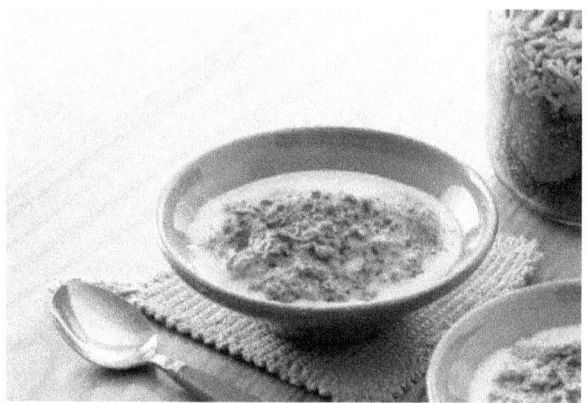

Serves 1

Ingredients

- 1 tablespoon flax seeds
- 1 cup non-dairy milk of your choice
- 1 tablespoon chia seeds
- Salt to taste
- 1 tablespoon sunflower seeds

Method

Set your stove to Med-High and mix the ingredients together into a smaller-sized saucepan. Let the mixture come to a boil and then reduce the heat. Allow it to simmer until as thick as you like. Serve with the milk of your choice or farm butter. Top with fresh fruit.

13. Simple Egg Mayo

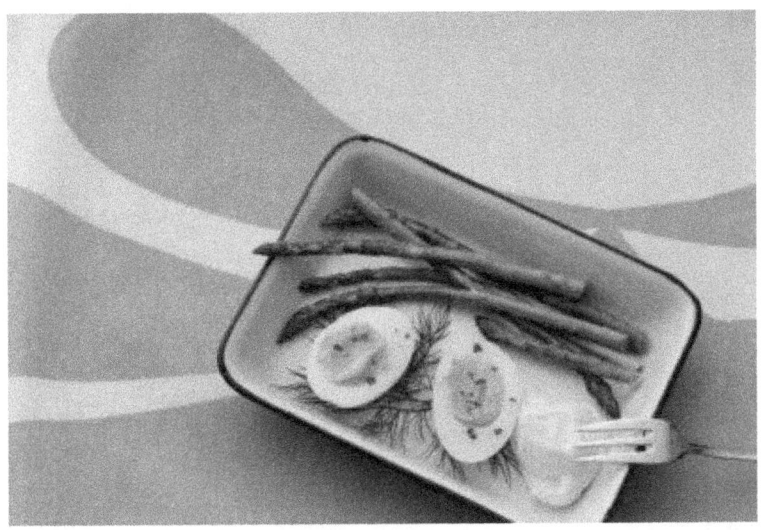

Serves 4

Ingredients

- Asparagus or avocado
- 8 tablespoons mayo
- 8 eggs

Method

Hard boil the eggs. (Around 8-10 minutes or so.) Let them cool down and peel. Halve the eggs. If using asparagus, cook until just done. If using avocado, remove the pit, peel and slice. Serve the eggs on a bed of asparagus/ avocado, topped with mayo.

14. Classic Bacon and Eggs

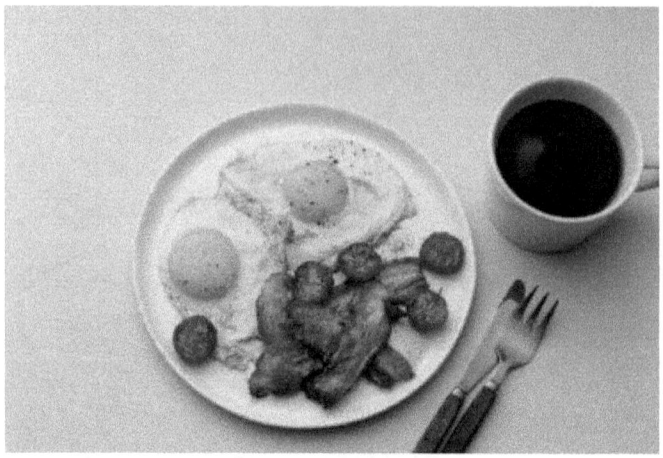

Serves 4

Ingredients

- ⅓ pound bacon, sliced into rashers
- 8 eggs
- Freshly picked parsley
- Cherry or Roma tomatoes

Method

Set the stove to Med-High and cook the bacon until it becomes crisp. Set to one side and keep it warm. Using the same pan, fry up the eggs until done to your liking. Halve the tomatoes and fry them. Season to taste and serve with the bacon, topped with the parsley.

15. No Dairy Latte

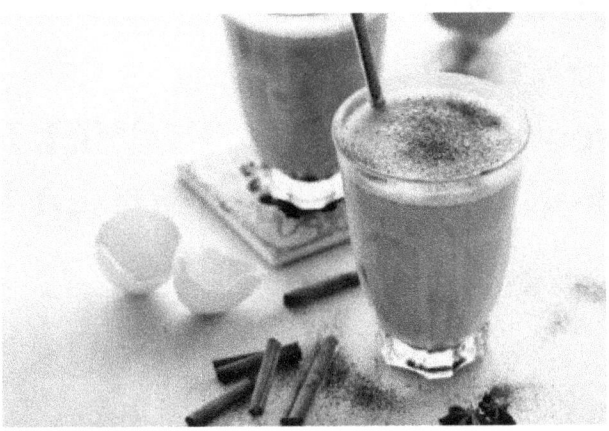

Serves 1

Ingredients

- 2 tablespoons coconut oil
- 2 eggs
- 1 2/3 cups boiling water
- 1 teaspoon pumpkin pie spice or powdered ginger
- 1 pinch vanilla essence

Method

Mix all the ingredients together using a blender and drink straight away.

Once again, thank you for reading this book, and I hope you're getting a lot of valuable information. I would greatly appreciate it if you could take 30 seconds to leave me a review for this book on Amazon.com.

Did You Know You Are MOST Likely Burning Fat Too SLOW?

Discover The Most POWERFUL Method to Start Burning Fat Up to 400% Faster!

For this month only, you can get Bruce's best-selling & most popular book absolutely free – *The Most Powerful Method to Burn Fat Up to 400% Faster!*

Get Your FREE Copy Here:
TopFitnessAdvice.com/Download

Discover exactly what you need to do to **put your metabolism into hyperdrive** and have your **fat melt away effortlessly**. And learn the biological "hacks" that have been scientifically proven to **boost the rate that your body burns fat by up to 400%.** With this book, readers were able to reach their fitness goals significantly quicker, so it's highly recommended that you get this book, especially while it's free!

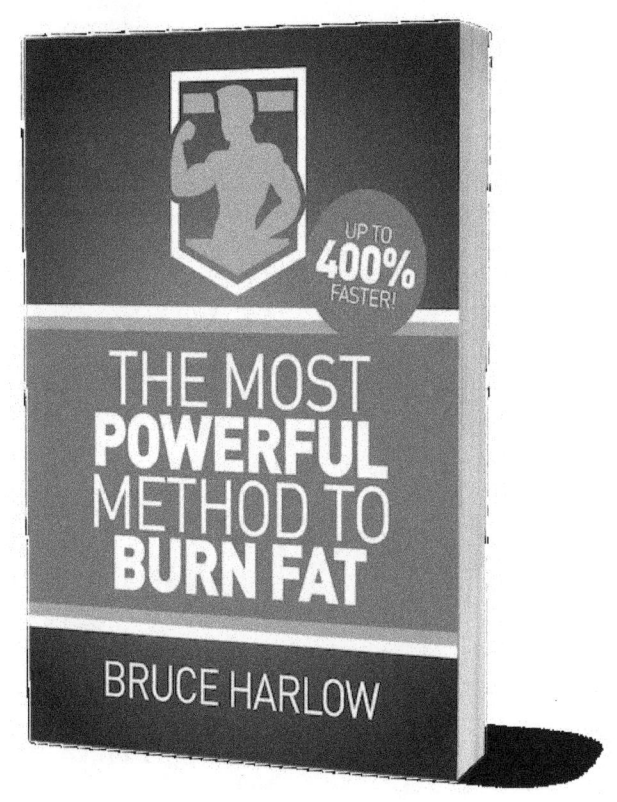

Get Your FREE Copy Here:

TopFitnessAdvice.com/Download

Chapter 2

Lunch

1. Veggie and Sausage Gratin

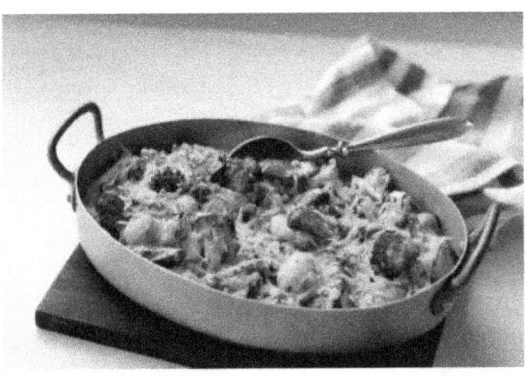

Serves 4

Ingredients

- 1 leek
- 1 pound sausages, cooked ahead of time
- 1 mild onion
- ½ pound cauliflower, chopped into florets
- 1 pound broccoli, chopped into florets
- 2 tablespoons Dijon mustard
- 4¼ ounces of Cheddar, grated
- 1 cup sour cream
- 1¾ ounces of farm butter
- Seasoning to taste
- 4 tablespoons freshly picked thyme, finely chopped

Method

Set your oven at 450. Chop up the onion and the leek roughly. Chop up the sausages into bite-sized bits. Cut up the sausages into bite-sized pieces. Set your stove to Med-High and melt the farm butter in a heavy-based frying pan.

Fry all the veggies until softened. Grease an oven-proof dish and layer the veggies and onion mix into it. Mix together the cream and the mustard and put it on top of the veggies. Stir in the sausage and season to taste. Top off with the thyme and the cheese. Put in the oven on the uppermost rack and cook for around 20 minutes.

2. Curried Cabbage

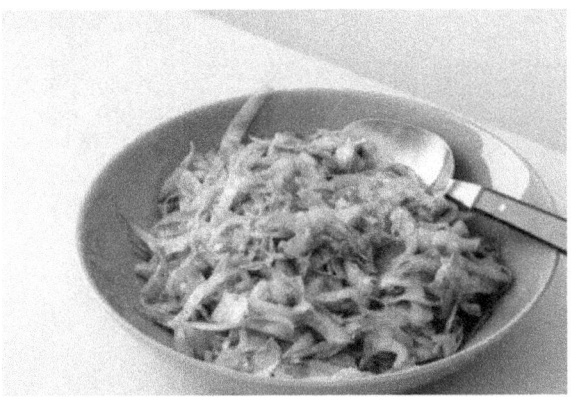

Serves 4

Ingredients

- 2 pounds cabbage, grated
- 3 tablespoons coconut oil
- 1 tablespoon red curry paste
- 1 tablespoon sesame oil
- 1 teaspoon table salt

Method

Set your stove to Med-High. Melt your coconut oil, stir in the curry paste and then put the cabbage and stir well. Cook until the cabbage starts to brown and caramelize but still has some crunch. Season as required and stir the sesame oil through. Fry for a couple of minutes.

3. Sausage and Cabbage

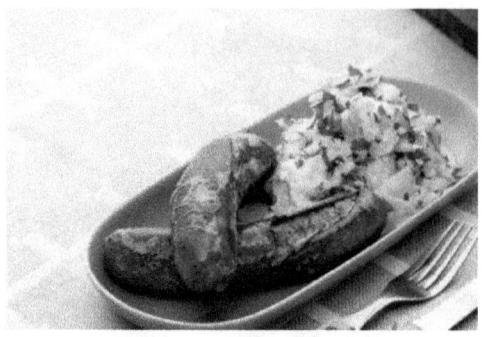

Serves 4

Ingredients

- 2 tablespoons farm butter
- 1½ pounds sausages of your choice

Ingredients for the Cabbage

- 2 ounces of farm butter
- 1½ pounds cabbage
- Seasoning to taste
- ½ lemon, the zest
- 1¼ cups double cream
- 8 tablespoons freshly picked parsley, chopped up nice and finely

Method

Set your stove to Medium and fry the sausages in the butter as you normally would. While the sausages are cooking, get another large frying pan ready to cook the cabbage. Set the stove to Med-High and melt the butter. Stir in the cabbage, making sure it is coated with the butter and fry until it starts to brown and caramelize.

Season to taste and stir in the cream. Reduce the heat to Low and cook, stirring often, until the cream reduces by half. Stir in the zest and parsley just before you serve the food.

4. Spicy Chicken and Rutabaga Bake

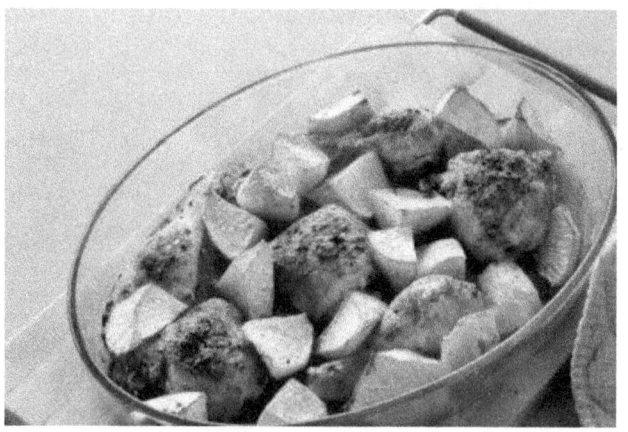

Serves 4-6

Ingredients

- 2 pounds rutabaga
- 2 pounds chicken thighs or drumsticks
- 1 cup mayo
- 4¼ ounces of farm butter
- Seasoning to taste
- 1 tablespoon powdered paprika

Method

Set your oven at 400. Grease and oven-proof dish and put the chicken into it in a single layer. Peel and cube the rutabaga into pieces that are a similar size to the chicken. Put in between the chicken pieces and season to taste. Sprinkle the paprika over the top.

Divide the butter up and place on top of the chicken and rutabaga – divide them as evenly as you can. Put into the oven and cook for about 40 minutes or until the chicken is cooked throughout. Serve with the mayo on the side.

5. Garlic Roast Chicken

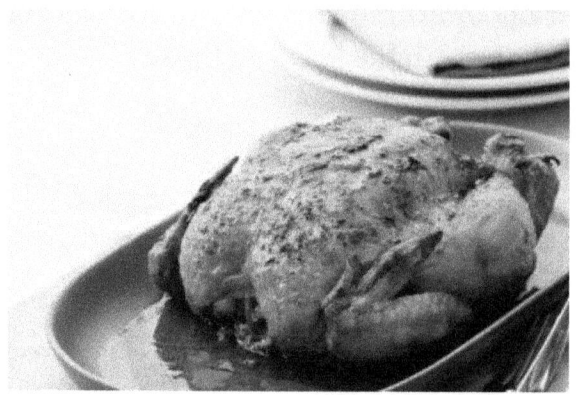

Serves 4

Ingredients

- 2 teaspoons table salt
- 1 chicken, a whole bird
- ½ teaspoon powdered black pepper
- 2 garlic cloves, crushed
- 1/3 pound farm butter

Method

Set your oven at 400. Clean the chicken and season to taste. Grease an oven-proof dish and place the chicken in it, with the breast facing up. Set your stove to Medium.

Using a small pan/ pot, melt the butter. Add the garlic and cook it for about a minute or two. Pour it over the chicken, trying to distribute it as evenly as possible.

Place on one of the lower racks of your oven and cook for a minimum of an hour, depending on how big the chicken is, basting every so often with the juice in the pan.

Your meat thermometer should reach 180 if the chicken is cooked. Alternatively, check that the juices run clear when you poke a whole into the thickest part of the chicken.

6. Leek and Broccoli Soup

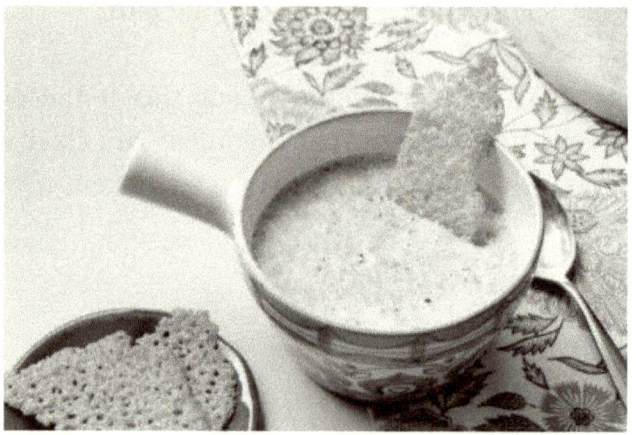

Serves 4

Ingredients

- 2 or 3 pounds of broccoli
- 1 leek
- ½ pound cream cheese
- 3 ounces of farm butter
- 3¼ cups water
- 2 tablespoons freshly picked basil, chopped
- Seasoning to taste
- ½ garlic clove

Ingredients for Cheese "Croutons"

- ½ teaspoon paprika powder
- 4¼ ounces of Cheddar

Method

Clean the leek and chop it up nice and finely – use the whole leek except for the roots. Remove the hard core of your broccoli and slice it up nice and finely. Break the florets up into small pieces and set to the side. Set the stove to High.

Put the broccoli and leek into a pot and cover with just enough water to submerge it. Bring to the boil. Season to taste and cook until just done. The broccoli should have some crunch left. Drain the broccoli.

Mix together the butter, the seasoning, the basil and the cream cheese with the broccoli and blend until it is smooth. If the soup is too thick, add water or some cream. Set your stove to Low and heat until warmed through.

Cheese Croutons: Set your oven at 400. Grate the Cheddar. Line a baking sheet with baking powder. Place mounds of the cheese onto the sheet. Season with paprika if you like. Place in the oven and cook for a few minutes until done.

7. Baked Eggs

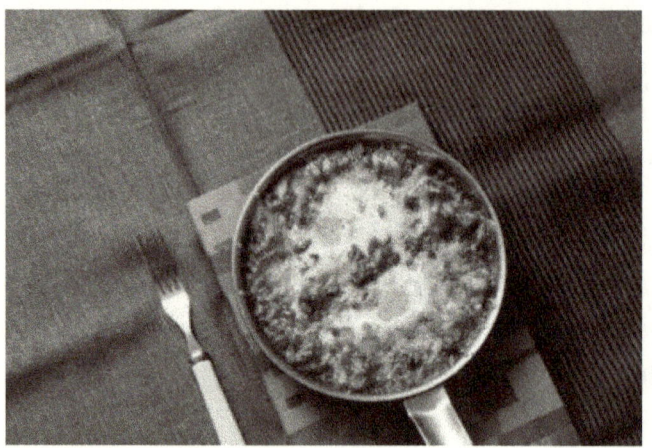

Serves 2

Ingredients

- 3½ ounces of beef mince, pre-cooked
- 2 ounces of cheese, grated
- 2 eggs

Method

Set your oven at 400. Grease a small oven-proof dish and spoon in the beef mince. Create two wells for the eggs and crack them into the well. Sprinkle the cheese over the top. Put in the oven and cook for around 15 minutes or until the eggs are done.

8. Creamy Turkey

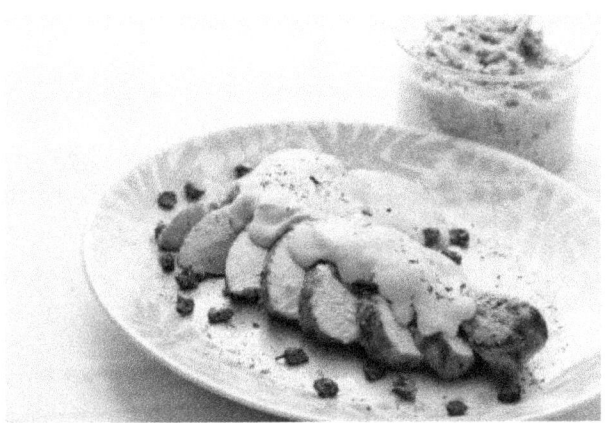

Serves 4

Ingredients

- 2 tablespoons farm butter
- 1 1/3 pounds turkey breast
- 2 cups sour cream
- Seasoning to taste
- 7 ounces of cream cheese
- 1 tablespoon soy sauce - optional
- 6 3/4 tablespoons small capers

Method

Set your oven at 350. Set your stove to Med-High. Melt the farm butter in a heavy-based frying pan. Brown the turkey in the butter. Season to taste. Grease and oven-proof dish and put the turkey into it. Cook until done.

When the turkey is just about done, put the sour cream into the frying pan and stir well. Reduce the heat to Low and allow the mixture to simmer until it is nice and thick. Adjust the seasoning as needed.

Add the soy sauce if you are using it. Set aside to keep warm. Set the stove to High and coat a little saucepan with butter. Fry up your capers for a few minutes.

9. Baked Peppers

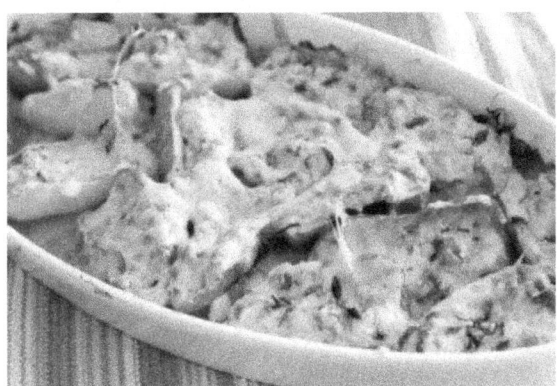

Serves 2

Ingredients

- ½ pound cream cheese
- ½ pound small bell peppers
- 1 ounces of chorizo, sliced up nice and finely
- 1 cup Cheddar, grated
- 2 tablespoons olive oil
- ½ – 1 tablespoon chipotle paste
- 1 tablespoon freshly picked cilantro, sliced up nice and finely

Method

Set your oven at 400°F. Halve the peppers lengthwise. Take out the seeds and the pepper's core. Chop up the sausage. Mix the cream cheese, the oil and the spices and mix well. Mix together with the sausage.

Grease an oven-proof dish and lay the peppers with the cut side up. Divide the cream cheese mixture between the peppers. Top with the Cheddar and bake for about 15 minutes.

10. Cheesy Veggies

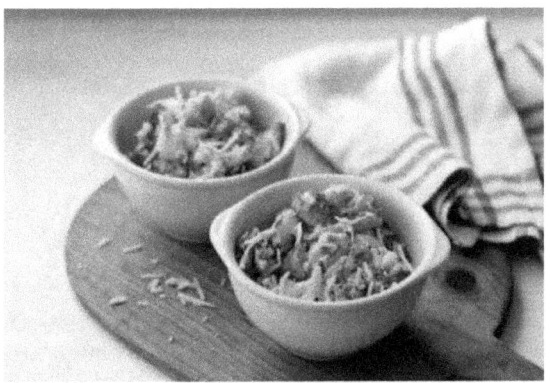

Serves 3-4

Ingredients

- 1 pound broccoli, finely chopped
- ½ pound cauliflower, finely chopped
- 3½ ounces of leeks, finely chopped
- 1¾ ounces of farm butter
- ⅓ pound Cheddar, grated
- 4 tablespoons sour cream
- Seasoning to taste
- 8 tablespoons freshly picked oregano, chopped up nice and finely

Method

Set your stove to Medium. Melt the farm butter in a large wok and add the veggies. Make sure they are coated with the butter and cook until done. Stir the cream and the cheese into the veggies and season as you like. Serve straight away.

11. Stuffed Chicken

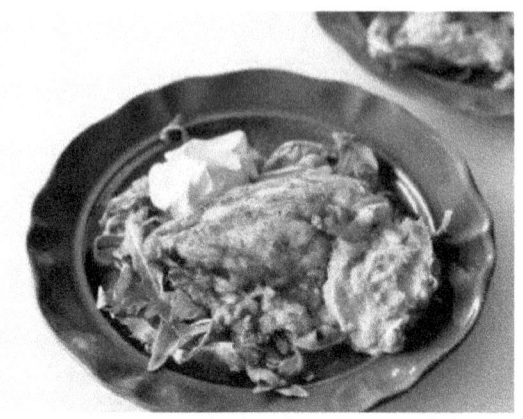

Serves 4

Ingredients

- 2 tablespoons olive oil
- 4 chicken breasts
- 1 mild bell pepper
- 2 tablespoons jalapeños, chopped up nice and finely
- 1 garlic clove
- ½ teaspoon powdered cumin
- ⅓ pound cheese, grated
- 3¼ ounces of cream cheese
- 4 tooth picks
- Seasoning to taste

Ingredients for Guacamole

- 1 – 2 garlic cloves
- 2 ripe avocados

- The juice of ½ lime
- ½ mild onion
- 3 tablespoons olive oil
- 5 ⅓ tablespoons freshly picked cilantro, chopped up nice and finely
- Seasoning to taste
- 1 diced tomato

To Serve

- ½ pound lettuce
- ⅔ cup sour cream

Method

Set your oven at 350. Chop up the garlic and the peppers nice and finely. Set your stove to Medium-High. Warm the oil in a heavy-based frying pan. Fry the peppers and the garlic until they are just starting to soften up. Put to one side and leave to cool. Mix the spices and the chili and both lots of cheese in a bowl. Add the pepper mixture.

Cut a pocket into each of the chicken breasts. Stuff each pocket with the mixture. Close off using a toothpick. Season to taste. Heat up some butter in a heavy-based frying pan. Fry the chicken until it is nicely browned all over.

Grease an oven-proof dish and put the chicken into it. Spoon any remaining pan juices over the top and put into the oven. Cook for 20-25 minutes or until the chicken is baked through. While that is cooking, make the Guacamole.

Guacamole: Peel and mash the avocados. Chop up the onion nice and finely and mix with the avocado. Add the lime juice and the remaining ingredients for the Guacamole and blend very well. Season to taste.

12. Cheeseburger with Mushrooms

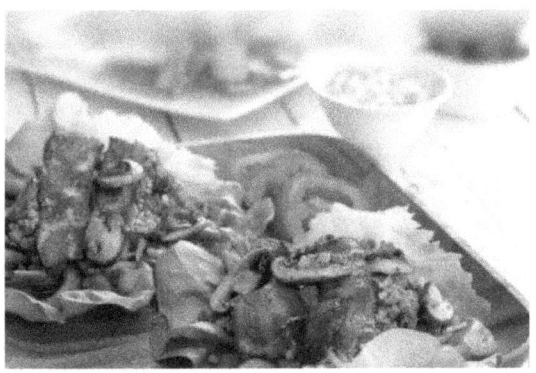

Serves 4

Ingredients

- 3½ ounces of mushrooms, thinly sliced
- 12 bacon rashers
- 1½ pounds beef, minced and formed into burger patties
- ¼ teaspoon pepper
- ½ teaspoon table salt
- 1 cup grated Cheddar
- Seasoning to taste
- 1 lettuce

Method

Set your stove to Med-High and heat up a frying pan. Fry the bacon until crisp. When done, drain on a piece of paper towel. Using the bacon fat, fry the mushrooms until done. Set aside where the mixture can be kept warm.

Using the same frying pan, cook the burger patties until done to your liking. Serve the patties on the lettuce, topped with the mushrooms and the cheese.

13. Mexican Cheeseburger

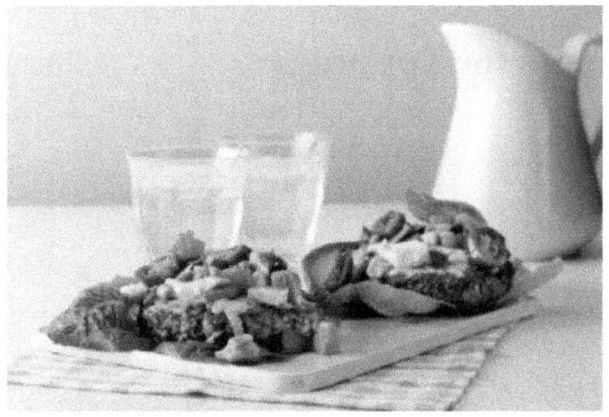

Serves 4

Ingredients

- 7 ounces of Cheddar, grated
- 1½ pounds beef, minced
- 2 teaspoons garlic powder
- 1 ounce of farm butter
- 2 teaspoons paprika
- 2 teaspoons onion powder
- 2 tablespoons freshly picked oregano, chopped up nice and finely

Ingredients for Salsa

- Fresh cilantro
- 2 scallions
- 2 tomatoes
- 1 avocado

- Salt
- 1 tablespoon olive oil

Ingredients for Toppings

- Jalapeños
- Cooked bacon
- Mayo
- Dijon mustard
- Lettuce
- Dill pickles

Method

Make the salsa by mixing all the ingredients together in a bowl. Set to one side. Now make the burgers. Mix together the beef and about half of the Cheddar. Season to taste.

Divide the mince mixture into four even-sized patties and fry until done to your liking. Top with the rest of the Cheddar. Serve on the lettuce and with the toppings of your choosing.

14. Jerk Chicken

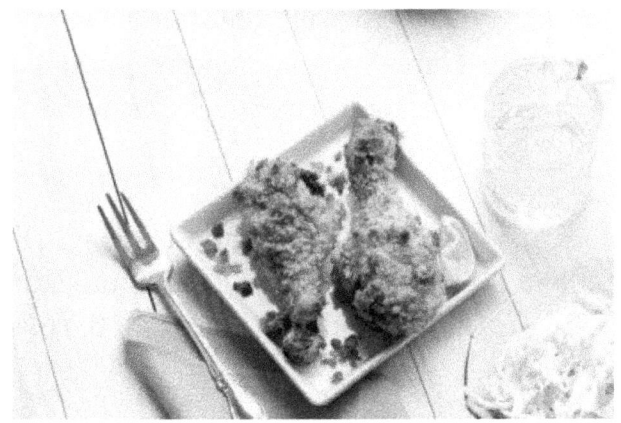

Serves 6-8

Ingredients

- 8 tablespoons sour cream
- 8 chicken drumsticks
- 2 tablespoons olive oil
- 1 teaspoon table salt
- 2 tablespoons jerk seasoning
- 1/3 pound pork rinds
- 4 tablespoons olive oil
- 3¼ ounces of desiccated coconut

Ingredients for Coleslaw

- Seasoning to taste
- 1 cup mayo
- 1 pound cabbage, grated

Method

Set your oven at 350. Mix the salt, the sour cream and the jerk seasoning. Place in a large bag and add the chicken. Shake the bag well so that the chicken is coated. Set aside for at least 20 minutes.

Remove the chicken and put in a different bag. Discard the marinade. Blend the pork rinds and coconut until crumbed. Put in the bag with the chicken and make sure that the pieces are all evenly coated as well.

Grease a broiler pan and put the chicken in it. Drizzle with the olive oil. Put in the oven and bake until the chicken is cooked through. It will take around 45 minutes, turning when about halfway through the cooking time.

In the meantime, make up the coleslaw. Blend all the coleslaw ingredients together and season to taste. Leave to one side for at least 15 minutes so that the flavors can develop.

15. Curried Chicken Pie

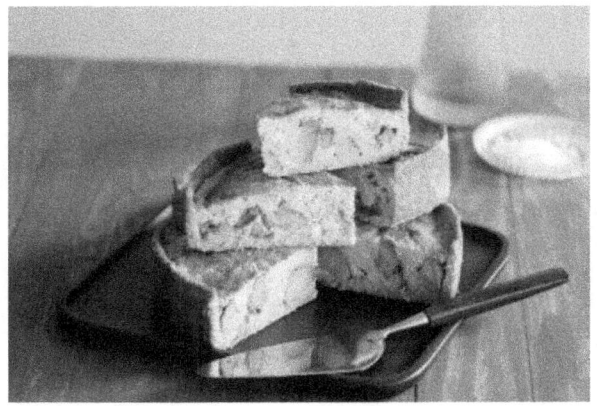

Serves 3-4

Ingredients for The Crust

- 4 tablespoons Sesame seeds
- ¾ cup almond flour
- 4 tablespoons coconut flour
- 1 teaspoon baking powder
- 1 tablespoon powdered psyllium husks
- 4 tablespoons water
- 1 pinch salt
- 1 egg
- 3 tablespoons olive oil

Filling

- 1 cup mayo
- ⅔ pounds cooked chicken
- 3 eggs

- 1 teaspoon curry powder
- ½ bell pepper, chopped up nice and finely
- ½ teaspoon paprika powder
- ¼ teaspoon powdered black pepper
- 1¼ cups Cheddar, grated
- ½ teaspoon onion powder
- 8 tablespoons cream cheese

Method

Set your oven at 350. Mix up all of the crust ingredients so that you get a firm dough. Grease a 10-inch pie plate and line it with a piece of baking paper. Spread out the dough in the plate – make sure it covers the base and sides of your pie plate.

Place in the oven and cook for between 10 and 15 minutes. Blend all of the ingredients for the filling and scoop into the crust. Place in the oven and cook for about 40 minutes or until the pie is going golden.

16. Garlic Chicken

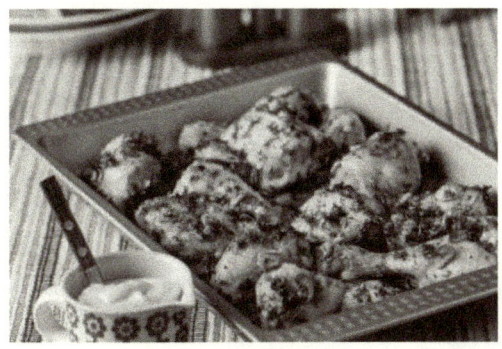

Serves 4

Ingredients

- 2 tablespoons olive oil
- 2¼ pounds chicken thighs
- 4 tablespoons farm butter
- 5 garlic cloves, sliced up nice and finely
- 8 tablespoons freshly picked parsley, chopped up nice and finely
- The juice of 1 lemon

Method

Set your oven at 450. Grease an oven-proof dish and put the chicken into it in a single layer. Season as required. Distribute the parsley and garlic over the top of the chicken. Mix the olive oil and lemon juice over the top.

Place the chicken in the oven and cook for about half an hour or so – or until the chicken is cooked throughout and crispy.

17. Caesar Salad

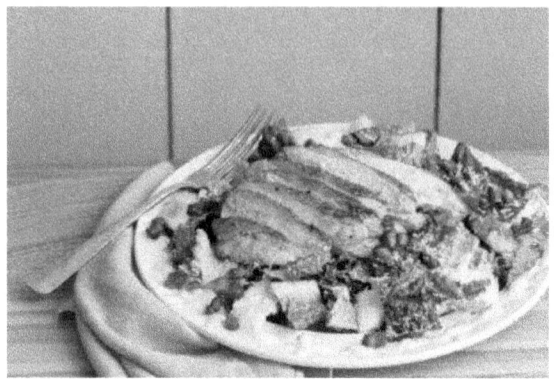

Serves 4

Ingredients

- 1 tablespoon olive oil
- 2/3 pound chicken breasts
- Seasoning to taste
- 1¾ ounces of fresh Parmesan, grated
- ½ Romaine lettuce
- 1/3 pound bacon

Dressing

- 1 tablespoon Dijon mustard
- ½ cup mayo
- The zest and juice of ½ a lemon
- 1 – 2 tablespoons anchovies, chopped up nice and finely
- 2 tablespoons fresh Parmesan, grated
- Seasoning to taste

Method

Start by making the dressing. Mix all the ingredients well and then mix so that the flavors can develop. Set your oven at 400°.

Grease an oven-proof dish and put the chicken into it in a single layer. Season to taste and drizzle with the olive oil. Place the chicken into the oven and cook until done throughout – about half an hour.

Set your stove to Med-High and fry up the bacon until it becomes crispy. Cut up the lettuce into bite-sized pieces and plate it. Serve the chicken on top. Top the chicken with the bacon and the rest of the Parmesan and then add your dressing.

Enjoying this book?

Check out our other best sellers!

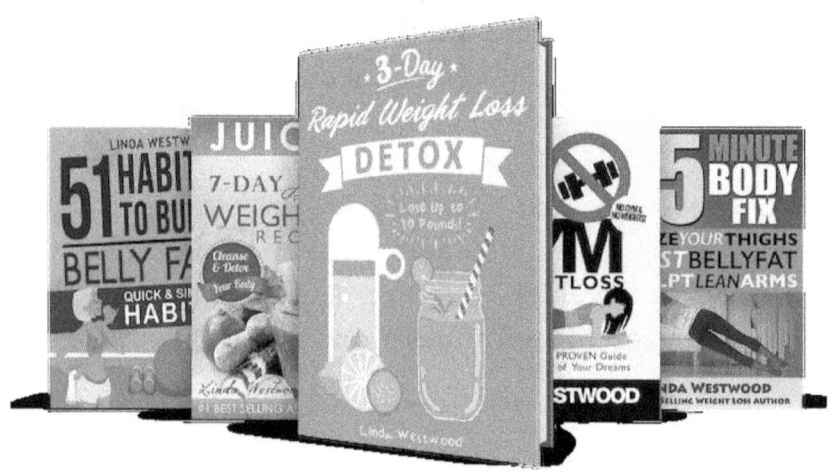

Get your next book on sale here:

TopFitnessAdvice.com/go/books

18. Chicken with Toasty Vegetables

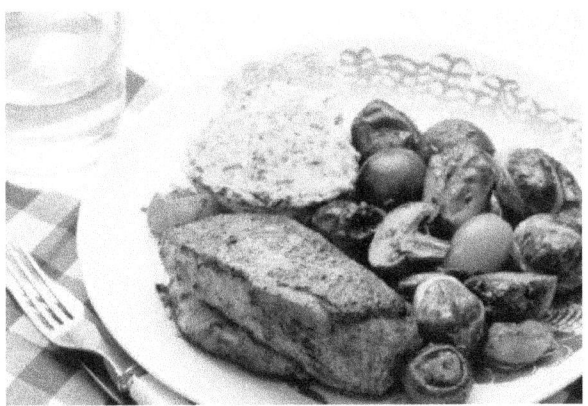

Serves 4

Ingredients

- ½ pound cherry tomatoes
- 1 pound Brussels sprouts
- ½ pound mushrooms
- ½ teaspoon powdered black pepper
- 1 teaspoon table salt
- 1 teaspoon dried rosemary

Ingredients for the Chicken

- 1 ounces of farm butter
- 8 tablespoons olive oil
- 4 chicken breasts
- 4¼ ounces of herb farm butter, to serve over the veggies

Method

Set your oven at 400. Grease an oven proof dish and add the veggies in a single layer. Season to taste and add the spices. Drizzle the olive oil over the top and mix well. Place in the oven for about half an hour or until the veggies are done.

Set the stove to Medium. Melt the butter in a large, heavy-based frying pan. Add the oil and warm it up. Season to taste and then cook the chicken until done. Serve with the veggies.

19. Herbed Chicken Breast

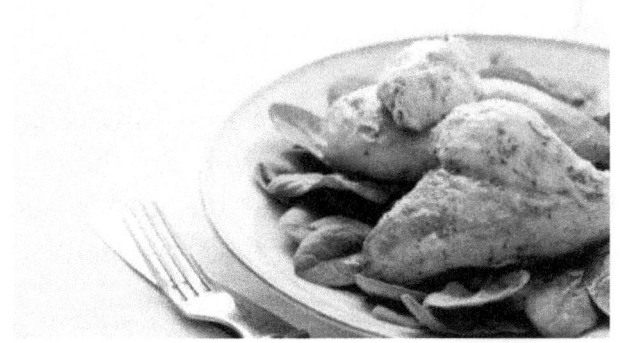

Serves 4

Ingredients

- 1 ounce of farm butter
- Seasoning to taste
- 4 chicken breasts

Ingredients for Herbed Farm Butter

- 1 garlic clove, crushed
- 1/3 pound farm butter, softened
- ½ teaspoon garlic powder
- 1 teaspoon lemon juice
- 4 tablespoons freshly picked parsley, chopped up nice and finely
- ½ teaspoon table salt
- ½ pound leafy greens of your choice

Method

Prepare the greens of your choice as you normally would. Next make the herbed butter. Mix the ingredients for the butter carefully until they are completely combined.

Move onto the chicken next. Season as required. Set your stove to Medium and melt the plain butter. Fry the chicken until cooked through and brown. Plate the greens and put the chicken on top. Serve with a pat of the herbed butter.

20. Skewered Chicken with Spinach Sides and Fries

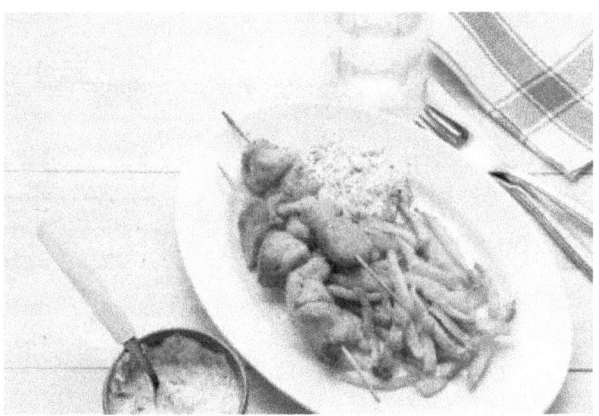

Serves 4

Ingredients

- 4 chicken breasts
- 4 – 8 wooden skewers
- ½ teaspoon table salt
- 2 tablespoons olive oil
- ¼ teaspoon powdered black pepper

Ingredients for Spinach Dip

- 2 ounces of spinach, chopped nice and finely
- 2 tablespoons olive oil
- 1 tablespoon dried dill
- 2 tablespoons dried parsley
- 1 teaspoon onion powder
- ¼ teaspoon powdered black pepper

- ½ teaspoon table salt
- 1 cup mayo
- 2 teaspoons lemon juice
- 4 tablespoons sour cream

Ingredients for the Fries

- ¼ powdered black pepper
- 2 tablespoons olive oil
- 1½ pounds root celery
- ½ teaspoon table salt

Method

Set your oven at 400. Start by making the dip. Mix all the dip ingredients together and stir well. Refrigerate. Cube the chicken into bite-sized pieces and put into a sealable bag. Add the oil and all the spices and shake. Ensure that all the chicken pieces are coated. Set aside to marinate for about 10 minutes.

While that is marinating, make the fries. Peel the celery root and cut into fries. Place in a clean bag and add the seasoning. Shake to coat. Grease a baking sheet and line with baking paper. Put the fries onto the baking sheet in a single layer and spread them out. Place them in the oven until done – around about 20 minutes or so.

Grease an oven-proof dish and put the chicken into it in a single layer. You can cook the chicken and the fries at the same time, keeping in mind that the chicken will take longer to get done.

21. BBQ Drumsticks with Spicy Aioli

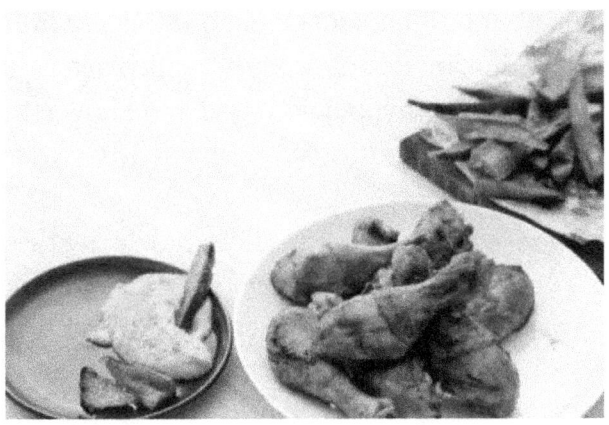

Serves 6

Ingredients

- Farm butter to coat the oven-proof dish with
- 2 tablespoons coconut oil
- 32 – 46 ounces of chicken drumsticks or chicken wings
- 2 tablespoons white wine vinegar
- 1 teaspoon table salt
- 1 tablespoon tomato paste
- 1 tablespoon tabasco
- 1 teaspoon paprika powder

Ingredients for Spicy Aioli

- 1 garlic clove, crushed
- 1 tablespoon powdered paprika
- 2/3 cup mayo

Method

Set your oven at 450. Place the chicken into a sealable bag. Mix together all the marinade ingredients and place in the bag as well. Make sure all the chicken is coated and allow it to marinate for a minimum of 10-15 minutes.

Grease an oven-proof dish. Put the chicken in the dish in a single layer. Put into the oven and cook for around half an hour to three quarters of an hour or until cooked through and crispy.

22. Cauliflower with Cheese

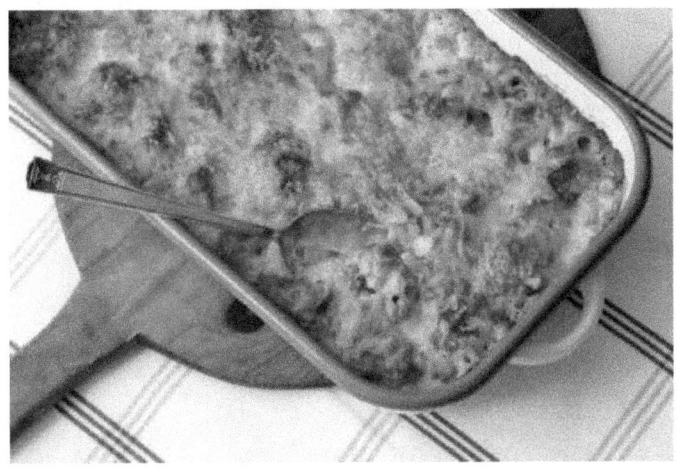

Serves 4

Ingredients

- 1 pound broccoli
- 1 cauliflower
- 7 ounces of plain cream cheese
- 1 2/3 cups Cheddar, grated
- 1¼ cups double cream
- 1¾ ounces of farm butter
- Seasoning to taste
- 1 – 2 teaspoons garlic powder

Method

Set your oven at 350. Boil the broccoli as normal and strain. Mix in the cream cheese, the cream and the garlic powder. Season to taste and blend until it is smooth. Grease a large oven-proof dish. Chop up the cauliflower into small pieces. Dot with the butter and pour the sauce over it. Put cheese on top and put it in the oven for about 40 minutes or till the cauliflower is cooked.

Chapter 3

Dinner

1. Italian Chicken and Noodles

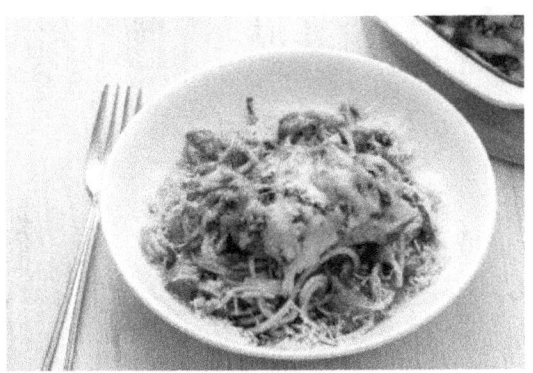

Serves 4

Ingredients

- 1/3 pound baby spinach
- 4 chicken breasts
- ½ pound ricotta cheese
- Fresh Parmesan, grated
- 2 ounces of farm butter
- 4 ounces of grated cheddar cheese
- Seasoning to taste

Ingredients for the Tomato Sauce

- 1 shallot
- 2 ounces of farm butter

- 2 garlic cloves
- 2 tablespoons tomato paste
- ½ tablespoon red wine vinegar
- 1 2/3 cups crushed tomatoes
- 1 teaspoon dried basil
- ½ teaspoon table salt
- pepper, to taste
- 1 teaspoon dried oregano

Ingredients for the Noodles

- 2 – 3 zucchinis

Method

Set your oven at 400. Set your stove to Medium-High. Put a little farm butter into a frying pan and cook the spinach until wilted. Season as required. Remove from the stove and mix in with the ricotta.

Cut the chicken lengthwise without cutting it right through. Grease an oven-proof dish and put the chicken into it. Spoon the spinach mixture into the slits you cut in the chicken. Put the Parmesan over the top. Finish off with the farm butter. Place in the oven for around half an hour or until the chicken is done.

In the meantime, make the tomato sauce. Chop up the garlic and shallots nice and finely. Set your stove to Med-High. Put the farm butter into a frying pan and add the garlic and shallots. Stir in the vinegar, tomatoes and tomato paste. Bring the mixture to a boil.

Stir in the herbs and reduce the heat to Low. Cook for 15 minutes. Make the zucchini into noodles by putting it through a spiralizer or by cutting the zucchini into thin noodles. Stir into the tomato sauce.

2. Roasted Salmon

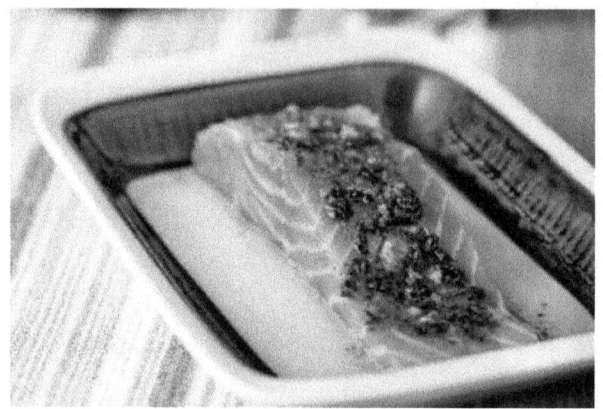

Serves 4

Ingredients

- Seasoning to taste
- 1¾ ounces of green pesto
- 2 pounds salmon

Ingredients for the Sauce

- 8 tablespoons Greek yogurt
- 1 cup mayo
- 1¾ ounces of green pesto
- Seasoning to taste

Method

Set your oven at 400. Grease an oven-proof dish and put the salmon into it, with the skin facing down. Put the pesto onto the salmon and spread it out evenly. Season as required. Put in the oven and cook for around half an hour or until the salmon is cooked. While that is cooking, mix together the ingredients for the sauce.

3. Cheese Bake

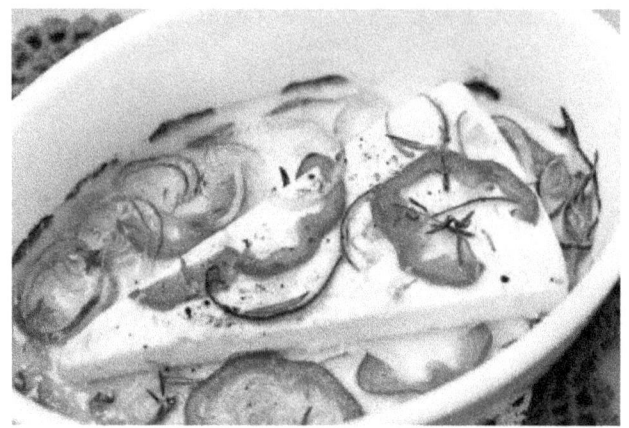

Serves 4

Ingredients

- 2 tablespoons olive oil
- ½ pound feta cheese or halloumi cheese
- 1 pinch chili flakes
- ¼ red onion, thinly sliced
- ¼ red bell pepper, thinly sliced

Method

Set your oven at 400. Grease an oven-proof dish. Put the cheese into the dish. Place the peppers and onions on the top of it. Sprinkle the spices and the oil over the top. Cook for 20-25 minutes or until the veggies are done.

4. Savory Pancakes

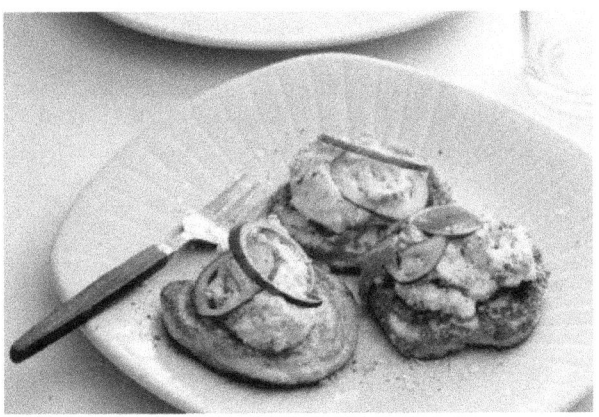

Serves 4

Ingredients

- 8¾ ounces of cottage cheese
- 5 eggs
- 1 pinch salt
- Farm butter
- 1 tablespoon powdered psyllium husks

Ingredients for the Topping

- 2 tablespoons green pesto
- ½ pound cream cheese
- ½ red onion, thinly sliced
- 2 tablespoons olive oil
- Powdered black pepper
- Table salt

Method

Start by making the topping. Mix together the oil, the pesto and the cream cheese. Put to one side. Now you can make the pancakes. Mix together the cottage cheese, psyllium powder, eggs and the salt until they are smooth. Set aside for 10 minutes so it can thicken.

Set your stove to Medium. Melt the farm butter in a heavy-based frying pan. When the butter has melted, drop spoonfuls of the batter into the pan and fry until done on both sides. Spoon the filling onto the pancakes and serve.

5. Halloumi Burger

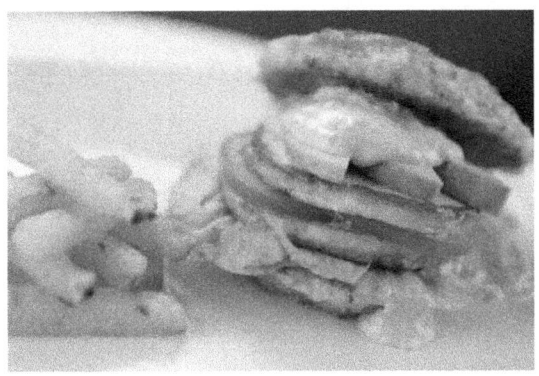

Serves 4

Ingredients for the Halloumi Burger

- Coconut oil
- 14 ounces of halloumi cheese
- 4 leaves of iceberg lettuce
- 1 avocado
- 1 tomato
- 6¾ tablespoons mayo
- 6¾ tablespoons sour cream
- 6¾ tablespoons ajvar relish
- 6¾ tablespoons coconut oil
- ½ rutabaga

Ingredients for the Cheesy Bread

- 1½ tablespoons powdered psyllium husks
- 4 eggs
- 2 teaspoons baking powder

- 2 cups Cheddar, grated
- 2 tablespoons chia seeds

Ingredients for the Toppings

- Table salt
- Poppy seeds

Method

Set your oven at 450. Peel the rutabaga and chop it into fries. Set your stove to Med-High. Place the rutabaga into a pot and cover it with water. Season to taste and boil for a few minutes. Drain the rutabaga well.

Melt the oil and pour over the fries. Make sure that the fries are completed coated. Season to taste. Grease a large baking sheet and lay the strips out on it in a single layer. Put in the oven and cook it until the chips start to go brown.

Mix together the relish, mayo and sour cream and put to one side. Make the bread next. Set your oven at 400. Whisk the eggs until they are fluffy. Mix together the dry ingredients. Mix in the cheese and then the eggs until the dough is smooth. Set aside for around 10 minutes.

Divide the batter into 8 equal portions. Place in the center of your oven and cook for about 10-15 minutes or until they have started to turn brown. Set your stove to Med-High. Grease a frying pan and cook the Halloumi until softens up. Assemble the burgers, adding in the toppings of your choice.

6. Eggplant Gratin

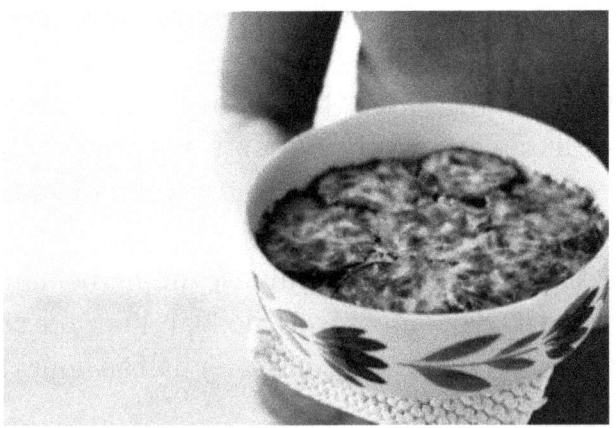

Serves 4

Ingredients

- 2 mild onions
- 2 pounds eggplants
- 2 tablespoons farm butter
- 1 tablespoon dried mint
- 1/3 pound feta cheese
- Seasoning to taste
- 6¾ tablespoons freshly picked parsley, chopped up nice and finely
- ¾ cup double cream
- 6¾ tablespoons Cheddar, grated

Method

Set your oven to 400. Cut the eggplants until slices about half an inch thick. Brush each slice with olive oil and season on both sides. Grease an oven-proof dish and line with baking paper. Put into the oven and cook until they are soft and slightly colored.

While that is cooking, slice up the onion nice and finely. Set your stove to Medium. Place a little butter in a pan and fry the onions until they soften. Season to taste. Set the oven to 450.

Layer the eggplants the fried onions, the herbs and the feta. Finish off with a layer of feta and Cheddar. Pour the cream over the top and place it in the oven. Cook for half an hour until done.

7. Cauliflower Cheese "Sandwiches"

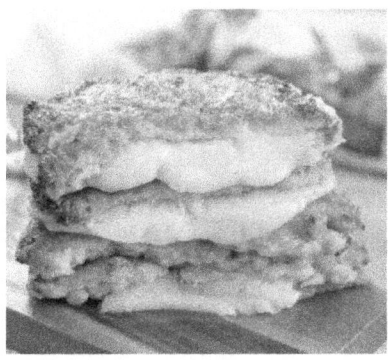

Serves 1

Ingredients

- 1 large egg
- 1 head of cauliflower, chopped into small bits
- 1/2 cup fresh Parmesan, grated
- 2 thick slices Cheddar
- 1 teaspoon Italian herb seasoning

Method

Set your oven at 450. Put the cauliflower in your food processor until it looks like small crumbs. Put into a big microwave dish and cover with cling wrap. Microwave for a couple of minutes on High.

Stir and put back in the microwave for 3 minutes. Repeat until the cauliflower is done. You want the cauliflower to look dry but to still retain some moisture.

Set it to one side so that it cools a bit and then stir in the Parmesan, seasoning and egg. Mix until it's smooth. Divide up the dough into four equally-sized portions.

Form into slices that look like bread and that are around a half inch thick. Place in the oven and cook for around 15 minutes or until done. Top two of the slices with the cheese and put the other slices on top. Place into the oven until the cheese melts.

8. Spinach Quiche

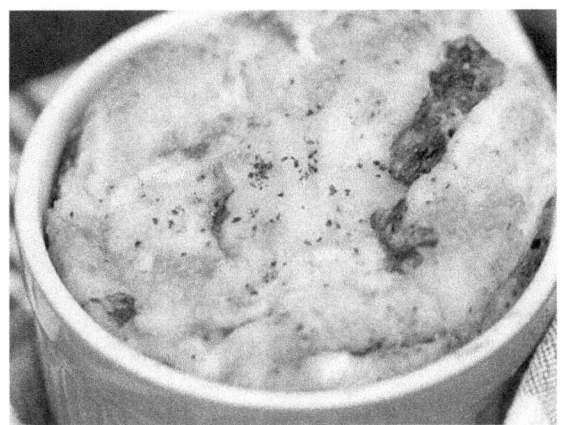

Serves 4

Ingredients

- 1 onion, chopped up nice and finely
- 1 tablespoon coconut oil
- ⅛ teaspoon black pepper
- 1 package frozen spinach, thawed – take as much water out as possible
- 3 cups Cheddar
- 8 eggs, beaten
- ¼ teaspoon table salt

Method

Set your oven at 350. Grease a pie plate. Set your stove to Medium. Melt the coconut oil in a heavy-based pot. Cook the onions until they are soft.

Mix in the spinach. Cook until all the moisture has cooked away. Mix together the cheese, seasoning and the eggs. Stir in the spinach. Place it in the pie plate, put it in the oven and cook for half an hour.

9. Slow-Cooked Chicken

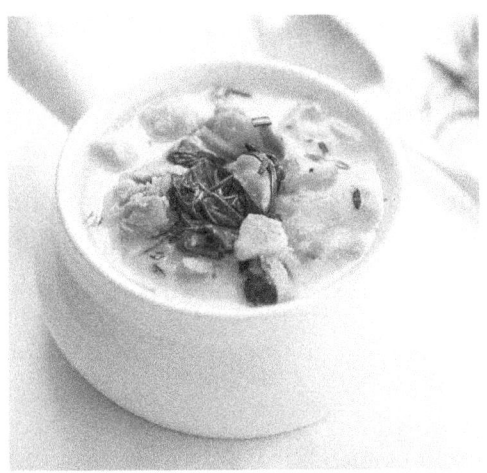

Serves 4

Ingredients

- 2 medium carrots, peeled and chopped up nice and finely
- 2 cups chicken stock
- 2 celery sticks, chopped up nice and finely
- 28 ounces chicken thigh fillets, cut into bite-sized pieces
- ½ onion (1/2 cup), chopped up nice and finely
- 1 sprig fresh rosemary
- ¼ teaspoon dried thyme
- 3 garlic cloves, crushed
- ½ teaspoon dried oregano
- Xanthan gum, to thicken the stew
- ½ cup heavy cream
- 1 cup fresh spinach
- Seasoning as required

Method

This is cooked in your slow cooker. Put the stock, herbs, carrots, onion, celery, and chicken into the slow cooker. Set the cooker to High and cook for 2 hours.

Season as required and then add the cream and spinach. Add the Xanthan gum, a pinch at a time until the stew is nice and thick. Stir well and then cook for a further 10 minutes.

10. Cheese Burgers with A Kick

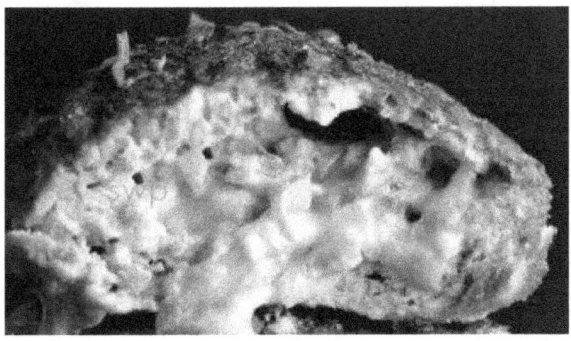

Makes 4 Patties

Ingredients

- Low carb bread
- 2 tablespoons onion, chopped up nice and finely
- 28 ounces of lean beef
- Salt & pepper to taste
- 2 ounces of Cheddar, grated
- 4 tablespoons cream cheese
- ¼ teaspoon garlic powder
- 1 tablespoon olive oil
- 1 fresh jalapeno pepper, chopped up nice and fine

Method

Set your grill to Medium. Mix together the Cheddar, the cream cheese, the chili and the garlic powder. In a second bowl, mix the meat and onion. Season to taste. Divide up into four evenly-sized patties.

Divide the cheese mixture between the patties and wrap the meat around them. Make sure that the filling is completely enclosed. Brush the patties with olive oil on both sides. Grill the burgers for around 6 minutes on each side or until they are cooked throughout.

11. Zucchini Loaf

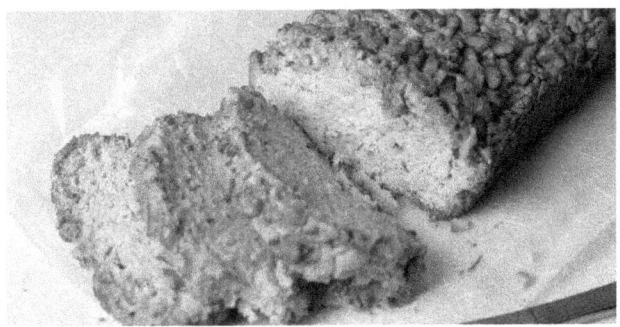

Serves 16

Ingredients

- ½ cup olive oil
- 3 large eggs
- 1 teaspoon vanilla essence
- 1 1/2 cups erythritol
- ½ cup chopped walnuts
- 2 1/2 cups almond flour
- ½ teaspoon table salt
- ¼ teaspoon ground ginger
- ½ teaspoon nutmeg
- 1 1/2 teaspoons baking powder
- 1 cup grated zucchini
- 1 teaspoon powdered cinnamon, powdered

Method

Set your oven at 350. Whisk the oil, vanilla essence and eggs. Put aside. In a clean bowl, combine all the dry ingredients and spices and put to one side. Put the zucchini into a clean tea towel and squeeze as much water as possible out.

Mix the zucchini in with the eggs and then blend into the dry ingredients. Grease a standard loaf pan and put the zucchini mixture. Top with the walnuts. Put in the oven for about an hour or until cooked throughout.

12. Mushroom Bites

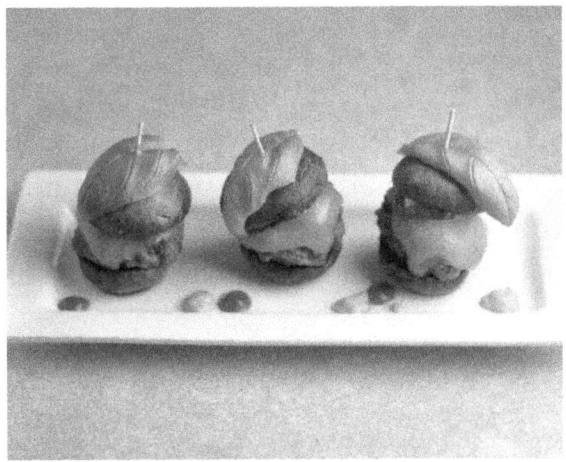

Makes 12

Ingredients

- 24 baby portabella mushrooms
- 1 pound beef, ground
- 4 slices Cheddar, cut into four equal parts
- 2 dill pickles, sliced
- 4 tablespoons onion, sliced into thin rings
- 2 tablespoons olive oil
- Sauces of your choosing
- 12 basil leaves
- Seasoning to taste

Method

Clean the mushrooms and take the stems out. Keep the stems for another day. Set your stove to Medium. Warm up a tablespoon of oil and then cook the mushrooms in it for a couple of minutes on each side. Place the mushrooms on paper towels to soak up excess moisture.

Season the beef to taste. Divide up the beef into 12 equally-sized balls. Flatten the balls. Set your stove to Medium. Heat up what is left of the oil and cook the patties for 3 minutes per side or until done to your liking. Use the mushrooms as "buns" and make up the "burgers" with the toppings that you like.

13. Tomato Soup

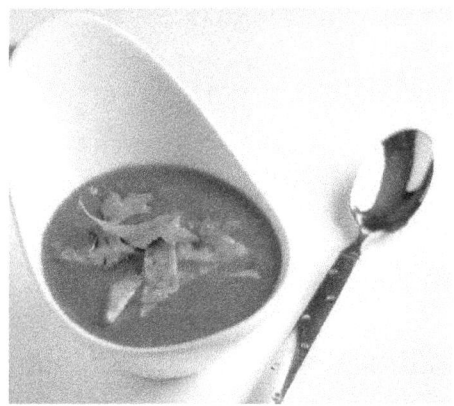

Serves 4

Ingredients

- 2 tablespoons onions, chopped up nice and finely
- 28 ounces of tomatoes, chopped up nice and finely
- 1 clove garlic, chopped up nice and finely
- 1 cup chicken broth
- 1/2 cup double cream
- 1/4 teaspoon garlic powder
- Seasoning to taste
- 2 tablespoons freshly picked parsley, chopped
- 1 cup Cheddar

Method

Set the oven at 350. Grease a baking tray and line it with baking paper. Place the Cheddar in piles on the baking sheet, leaving enough space between the piles so that there is space for the melted cheese to spread. Add a little garlic powder to each pile. Place in the oven and cook for about five minutes or until the cheese crisps a little.

Set your stove to Medium. Put the oil into a heavy-based saucepan and heat it up. Add the onions and the garlic. Fry until the onions have just softened. Stir in the tomatoes. Bring the liquid to the boil and then reduce the heat to Low. Cook for around 5 minutes.

Mix in the broth. Bring to the boil and simmer it for five more minutes. Add the cream and adjust the seasoning if necessary. Serve with the cheese chips you made and garnish with the parsley.

14. Beef Satay

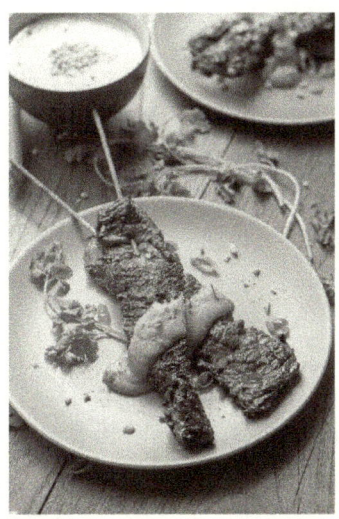

Serves 4

Ingredients for Beef Satay & Marinade

- 2 tablespoons fish sauce
- 1 pound skirt steak
- 2 tablespoons soy sauce
- 1/2 teaspoon ground coriander
- Sweetener to taste

Ingredients for Thai Peanut Sauce

- 1/3 cup whole fat coconut milk
- 1/4 cup smooth nut butter
- 1-2 teaspoons garlic chili sauce
- 1/2 teaspoon Thai red curry paste

Extras

- Foil
- Skewers that have been soaked in water for at least half an hour
- 1 tablespoon olive oil

Method

Beef Satay: Cut up the steak into strips. Mix together the soy sauce, sweetener and fish sauce. Coat the beef in the soy sauce mixture. Marinade it for about half an hour and then skewer the meat. Pre-heat your grill and make the sauce. Heat the nut butter in the microwave for about 10-15 seconds so that it is easier to blend.

Mix with the garlic chili sauce, the curry paste, and the sweetener. Whisk in the coconut milk. Coat the beef with some of the oil. Cover the end of the skewers with the foil. Grill the skewers until the meat is done to your liking.

Grill: Pour about 1 tablespoon of oil over the beef and coat all surfaces. Fold a piece of foil in half to be placed under the handles of the skewers while cooking on the grill.

Remove the beef from the marinade and place it on the grill for cooking. Line them up and place the foil under the handles. Grill on both sides until done - this depends on how thick your meat is and how hot your grill gets.

15. Alfredo for Vegans

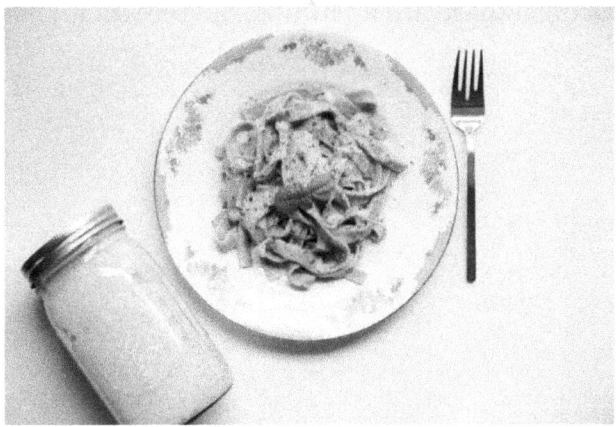

Serves 4

Ingredients

- 2 tablespoons olive oil
- 1 small head of cauliflower, chopped up nice and finely
- 2 cloves garlic, crushed
- 2¼ cup non-dairy milk
- 2 teaspoons pine nuts
- 2 teaspoons of oregano and basil
- Seasoning to taste
- ¼ cup plus 1 tablespoon nutritional yeast
- Juice of half a lemon

Method

Set the stove to Medium-High. Put the oil into a put and fry the pine nuts and garlic in it for a few minutes. Put the milk in and bring the mixture to the boil. Lower the heat Medium. Stir in the cauliflower with the spices. Cook till the cauliflower is done. Put the mixture into your blender and add the remaining ingredients until there are no lumps. Serve with low-carb pasta.

16. Hot Steak

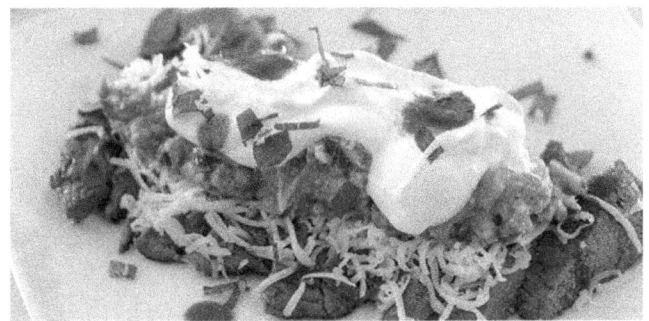

Serves 4

Ingredients

- Seasoning to taste
- 16 ounces of skirt steak
- Guacamole to serve with
- 1 splash of Tabasco Sauce
- 1 cup sour cream
- 4 ounces of pepper jack cheese
- 1 handful freshly cilantro, chopped up nice and finely

Method

Season your steak as you like. Set your stove to High and warm up a heavy-based pan. Brush the steak with oil and cook until it is done to your liking. Let the meat rest for about 5 minutes.

Slice the steak into manageable strips. Top with the cheese and some guacamole. Finish with a drop of Tabasco sauce and the sour cream. Use the cilantro as a garnish.

17. Greek Meatballs

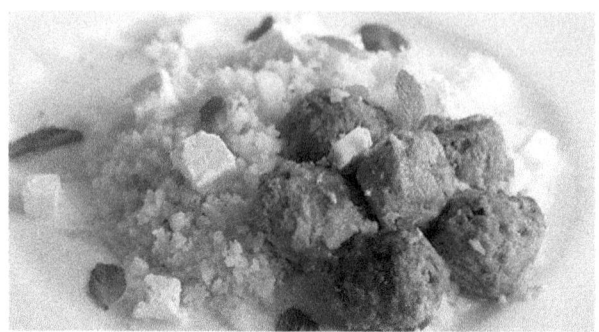

Servings 4

Ingredients for the Cauliflower Rice

- Seasoning as required
- ½ pound of cauliflower

Ingredients for the Meatballs

- 1 large egg
- 1 pound lamb, ground
- 1 teaspoon pepper
- 1 teaspoon salt
- 1 teaspoon garlic powder
- 1 teaspoon paprika
- 1 teaspoon fennel seed

Additional Ingredients

- 4 ounces of goat cheese
- ½ mild onion, chopped up nice and finely

- 2 tablespoon coconut oil
- A crushed garlic clove
- 1 tablespoon lemon zest
- 1 bunch fresh mint leaves, chopped nice and finely

Method

Start off by making the cauliflower rice. Pulse the cauliflower until it looks like rice. Boil the cauliflower until done. Put to one side. Mix together the eggs, spices and the lamb. Divide the mixture into 12 even-sized meatballs and put to one side.

Set your stove to Medium. Melt the coconut oil in a heavy-based pan and fry the onion. Cook until the onions soften. Stir in the garlic and cook for a minute or so.

Put the meatballs in the pan. Cook on all sides until the meat is done. Serve with the "rice" with mint, zest and the cheese.

18. Shrimp and Garlic Pasta

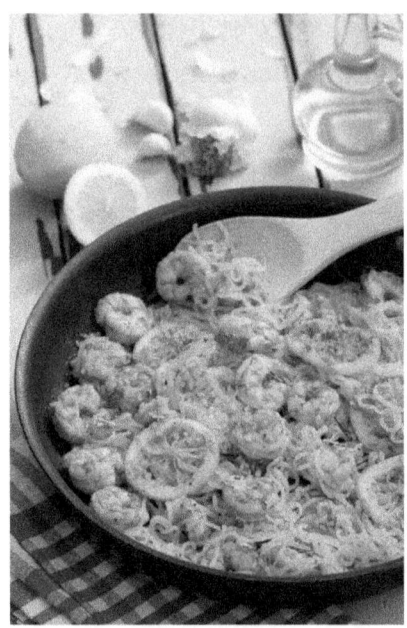

Servings 4

Ingredients

- Freshly picked basil, chopped up nice and finely
- 2 tablespoons farm butter
- 2 bags low-carb Angel Hair pasta
- 2 tablespoons olive oil
- 1/2 lemon
- 4 cloves garlic
- 1 pound large raw shrimp
- Seasoning to taste
- 1/2 teaspoon paprika

Method

Set your stove to Med-High. Melt the oil and the farm butter in a heavy-bottomed frying pan. Add the garlic to the pan and cook for about a minute. Chop the lemon into round slices.

Place the shrimp and lemon into the frying pan. Cook for around about 6 minutes, stirring often. Once the shrimps have finished cooking, stir in the pasta and season to taste. Add in the paprika. Cook the pasta according to the package instructions.

19. Chicken Thighs with Lemon and Rosemary

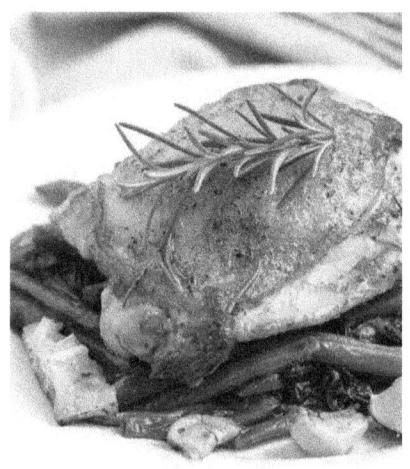

Serves 2

Ingredients

- 2 tablespoons farm butter
- Seasoning to taste
- 4 Chicken Thighs
- 1 Lemon
- 4 sprigs of fresh rosemary
- 2 cloves of garlic

Method

Set your oven at 400. Set the stove to High. Melt a little butter in a heavy-bottomed frying pan and put the chicken in it, with the skin side facing down. Cook until brown and flip them over.

Chop the lemons into quarters and squeeze the juice over the chicken pieces. Put the lemon pieces into the pan as well.

Chop the garlic up and put it into the frying pan. Add the rosemary as well. Transfer the mixture to an oven-proof dish and cook it for half an hour. Chop up some farm butter and put it out onto the chicken. Put it back in the oven for another 10 minutes.

20. Pork Loin with A Creamy Sauce

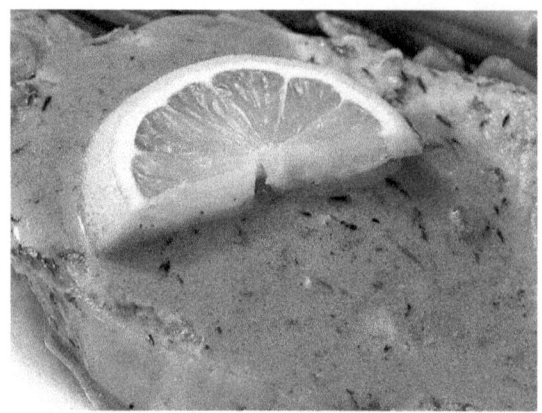

Serves 2

Ingredients for the Pork Loins

- 1 tablespoon table salt
- 4 4 ounces of pork loin
- 1 teaspoon black pepper
- 1 teaspoon thyme
- 1 teaspoon paprika

Ingredients for the Creamy Sauce

- 1/4 cup double cream
- 1/2 cup chicken stock
- 1 teaspoon apple cider vinegar
- 1 tablespoon mustard
- 1/2 lemon

Method

Pat the pork dry and then season as required with the paprika, thyme and salt. Set your stove to High. Grease a frying pan and brown the pork in it. Put them to the side where they can stay warm. Set your stove to Medium.

Using the same pan, mix together the vinegar, the cream and the chicken stock. Scrape the bottom of the pan so that all the leavings from the pork are incorporated into the sauce. Stir in the mustard and the lemon.

Place the pork into the sauce. Flip it to ensure both sides are coated. Cover the pan, leaving a small space for the steam to escape and cook for 10 minutes or until the pork is cooked through.

21. Meatballs A La Coconut

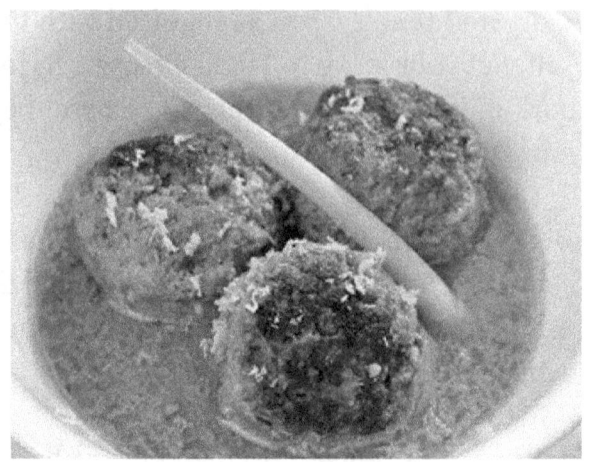

Serves 4

Ingredients for the Meatballs

- 1 pound beef, ground
- 1 tablespoon coconut oil
- 1 tablespoon table salt
- 1/2 onion
- 1/2 cup almond flour
- 4 cloves garlic
- 2 tablespoons non-dairy milk

Coconut Broth

- 1 cup broth
- 1 cup coconut milk
- 2 teaspoon coriander seeds
- lime zest

- 1 teaspoon powdered cinnamon
- 1 teaspoon turmeric
- 1 teaspoon crushed red pepper
- 1 inch fresh ginger
- 1 stalk lemongrass

Method

Set your stove to Med-High. Grease a pan and stir in the onions and garlic until they are soft. In the meantime, mix together the flour and milk, creating a smooth paste.

Mix the mince in with the paste and season to taste. Stir in the cooked garlic and onions. Divide the mixture up and roll into meatballs about two inches across.

Set your stove to Medium. Use some farm butter to coat the frying pan and then brown the meatballs on all sides. Leave the center of the frying pan clear so that you can put the spices in it. The spices will heat up and form a paste with the butter.

Once the meatballs are brown, add the broth and coconut milk. Stir well. Crush the lemongrass and put it into the soup. Add the ginger and let the mixture come to the boil. Reduce the heat to Low and cook for about 15 minutes or until the meatballs are properly cooked.

22. Thai Chicken Soup

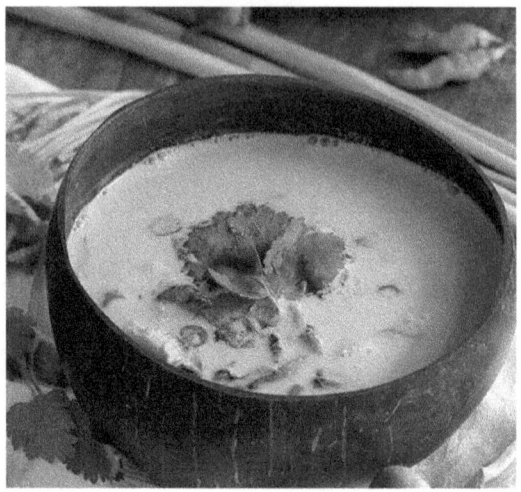

Serves 4

Ingredients

- 2 stalks lemongrass, crushed
- 6 cups chicken stock
- 10 lime leaves
- 1/2 teaspoon table salt
- 1 inch fresh ginger
- 1 pound boneless skinless chicken thighs
- 1.5 cups coconut cream
- 10 ounces of mushrooms of your choice
- 1 tablespoon fish sauce
- Cilantro, chopped up nice and fine, to taste
- 1 chili pepper if you like

Method

Set your stove to Med-High. Put the stock into a pot. Chop the lemongrass up and add to the stock. Stir in the lime leaves, salt and ginger. Bring to a boil and reduce the heat to Low. Cook for around 20 minutes. Strain out the solids.

Set the stove to Med-High. Now add in the chicken and the mushrooms and bring them to a boil. Reduce the heat to Low and cook for a further 20 minutes or until the chicken is done.

Shred the chicken and put it back into the soup. Add the fish sauce and some coconut cream and cook for about 5 minutes or until completely heated through.

Others who are considering purchasing this book would love to know what you think. If you could spare a few seconds, they would greatly appreciate reading an honest review from you. Simply visit the page on Amazon.com.

Chapter 4

Snacks

1. Cheese Puffs

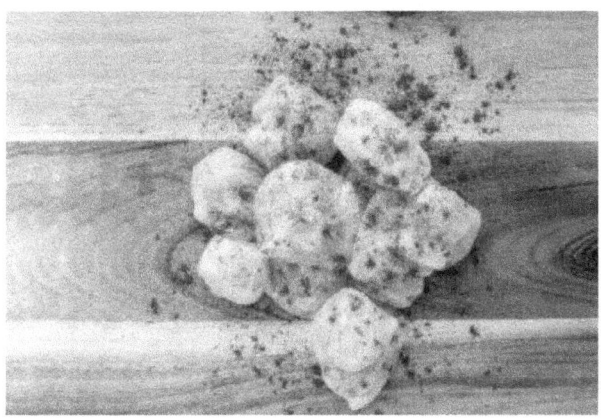

Serves 3

Ingredients

- Paprika
- 1/3 pound Brie

Method

Cut the white edge off the cheese and cut it into half-inch squares. Line a microwavable plate with baking paper. Lay out the cheese in a single layer and cook on high for around minute or two. Season with paprika and serve immediately.

2. Herbed Cream Cheese

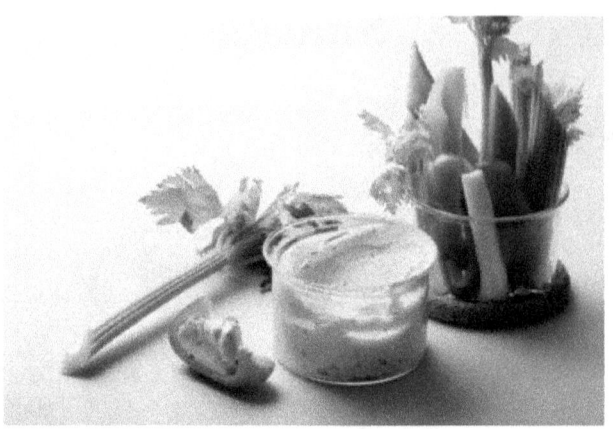

Serves 4

Ingredients

- 2 teaspoons olive oil
- ½ pound cream cheese
- 8 tablespoons freshly picked parsley, chopped up nice and finely
- The zest of ½ a lemon
- 1 garlic clove, crushed
- 4 celery stalks, or other fresh vegetables of your liking
- Seasoning to taste

Method

This is best if made the night before you want to use it to allow the flavors to develop. Mix all of the ingredients together and put in the refrigerator to set.

3. Bread Sticks

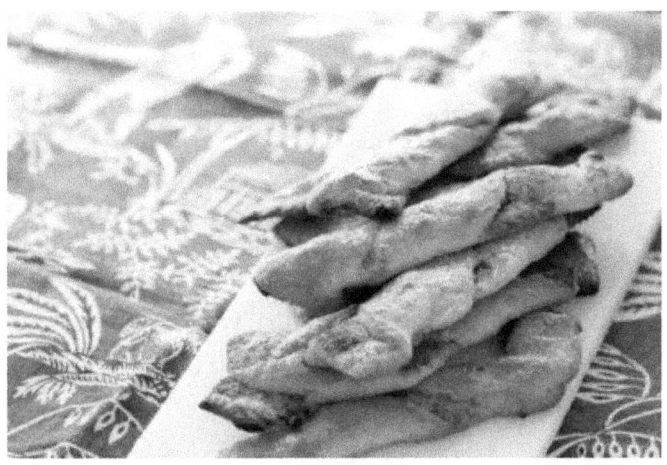

Serves 10

Ingredients

- 1 egg
- 4 tablespoons coconut flour
- 8 tablespoons almond flour
- ½ teaspoon table salt
- 1½ cups Cheddar, grated
- 1 teaspoon baking powder
- 2 2/3 ounces of farm butter
- 2 ounces of green pesto
- 1 egg

Method

Set your oven at 350. Mix together all dry ingredients. Set the stove to Low. Put the farm butter into a saucepan and melt it.

Mix the cheese in and cook until the cheese is melted. Beat one of the eggs and add it to the butter mixture.

Mix it into the dry ingredients to make a dough. Roll out the dough until it is about 1/5 of an inch thick. Line a baking sheet with baking paper.

Put the pesto over the top of the dough, evenly. Slice the dough into strips about an inch in width. Twist the dough and brush with the other beaten egg. Put into your oven and cook for around 15 minutes or until they are crisp and done.

4. Green Beans and Parmesan

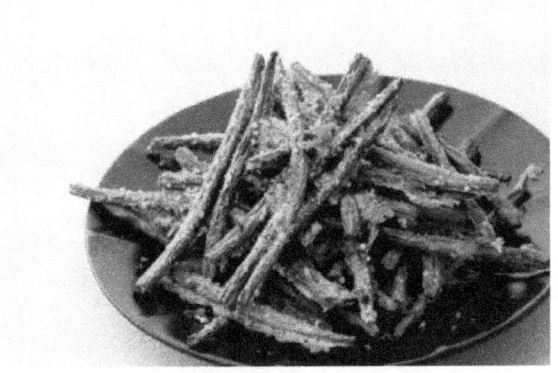

Serves 4

Ingredients

- 5 1/3 tablespoons fresh Parmesan, grated
- 2 tablespoons olive oil
- 1 egg
- 1 teaspoon onion powder
- 2 pinches pepper
- ½ teaspoon table salt
- 1 pound fresh green beans

Method

Set your oven at 450. Grease a baking tin and line it with parchment paper. Beat the eggs, spices and oil together. Trim the beans and coat them with the batter. Follow up with a coating of Parmesan. Lay the beans out on the baking tin and cook until the beans are cooked through.

5. Cabbage Comfort Food

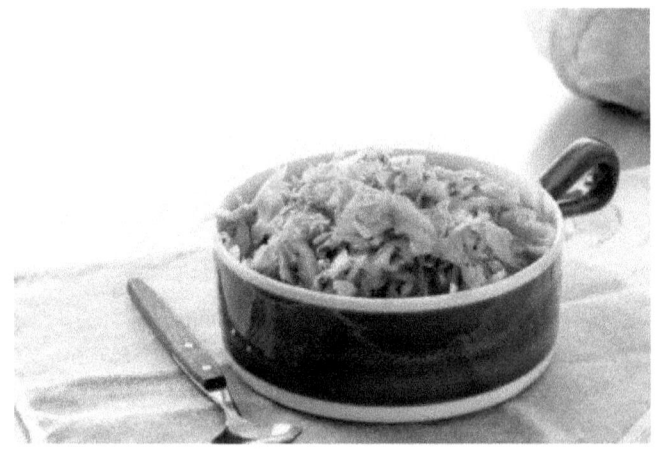

Serves 4

Ingredients

- Seasoning to taste
- 3½ ounces of farm butter
- 1½ pounds cabbage, grated

Method

Set your stove on Medium. Place the butter into a large frying pan and melt it. Add the cabbage and stir until completely coated. Season as you like and cook for about 15 minutes. The cabbage should be just cooked.

6. Cheese and Bacon Bites

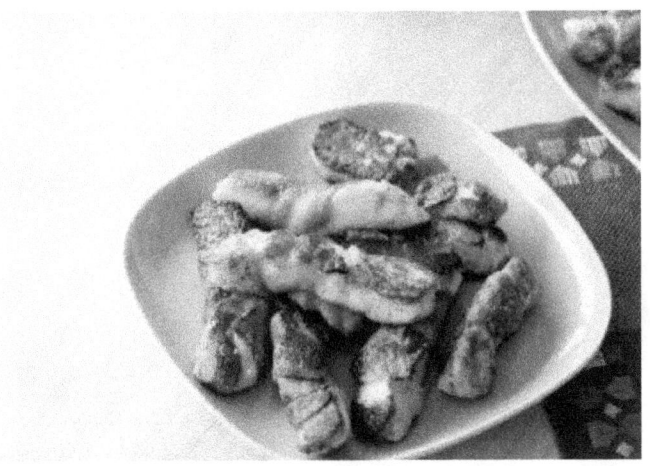

Serves 2

Ingredients

- ⅓ pound bacon, sliced into thin wafers.
- ½ pound halloumi cheese

Method

Set your oven at 450. Chop the halloumi into 8 sticks. Wrap the bacon around the cheese. Grease a baking sheet and line it with baking paper. Put the cheese sticks on the sheet and cook for around 5-7 minutes per side.

7. Tacos with A Twist

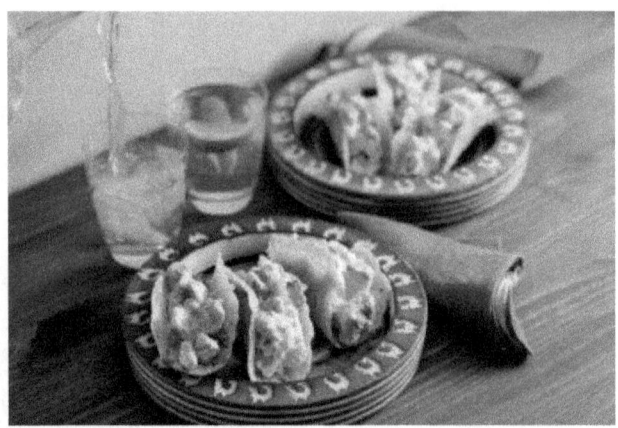

Serves 2

Ingredients for Taco Shells

- ½ teaspoon powdered cumin
- ½ pound Cheddar, grated

Ingredients for the Creamy Shrimp Filling

- 2 tablespoons coconut oil
- 2/3 pound cleaned shrimps, peeled
- 2 garlic cloves, chopped up nice and finely
- 1 cup mayo
- 1 red chili pepper, deseeded and chopped up nice and finely
- The juice of ½ lime
- 1 avocado, diced
- 4 tablespoons freshly picked cilantro, chopped up nice and finely

- Seasoning to taste
- 1 tomato, chopped up nice and finely

Method

Taco Shells: Set your oven at 400. Mix the cumin and the Cheddar. Line a baking sheet with baking paper. Divide the cheese up unto 8 different piles, leaving space in between each to allow the cheese to spread out. Cook for around 10 minutes or till the cheese bubbles and is crisp.

Take out of the oven and wait for about half a minute. Carefully shape the cheese tacos into a taco shape by draping them over a rack and leaving them to cool.

For the Filling: Set the stove to High. Put the coconut oil in a large frying pan and stir in the shrimp, chili and garlic. Season as required and cook the shrimp until they turn pink and are done. Mix everything else for the filling and stir in the shrimp. Serve in the taco shells.

8. Berry Dessert

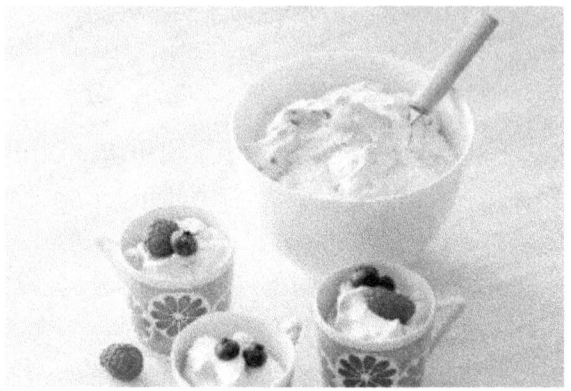

Serves 2

Ingredients

- 1¾ ounces of pecan nuts, chopped up nice and finely
- 3¼ ounces of mixed berries
- The zest of ½ lemon
- 2 cups double cream
- ¼ teaspoon vanilla essence

Method

Whip the cream until soft peaks form. Mix in the vanilla essence and the lemon zest gently. Put the nuts and berries in and store the mousse in the fridge for a few hours so that it can set.

I hope you have learned something from this book so far and would greatly appreciate it if you could leave an honest review on Amazon.com.

Did You Know You Are MOST Likely Burning Fat Too SLOW?

Discover The Most POWERFUL Method to Start Burning Fat Up to 400% Faster!

For this month only, you can get Bruce's best-selling & most popular book absolutely free – *The Most Powerful Method to Burn Fat Up to 400% Faster!*

Get Your FREE Copy Here:
TopFitnessAdvice.com/Download

Discover exactly what you need to do to **put your metabolism into hyperdrive** and have your **fat melt away effortlessly**. And learn the biological "hacks" that have been scientifically proven to **boost the rate that your body burns fat by up to 400%.** With this book, readers were able to reach their fitness goals significantly quicker, so it's highly recommended that you get this book, especially while it's free!

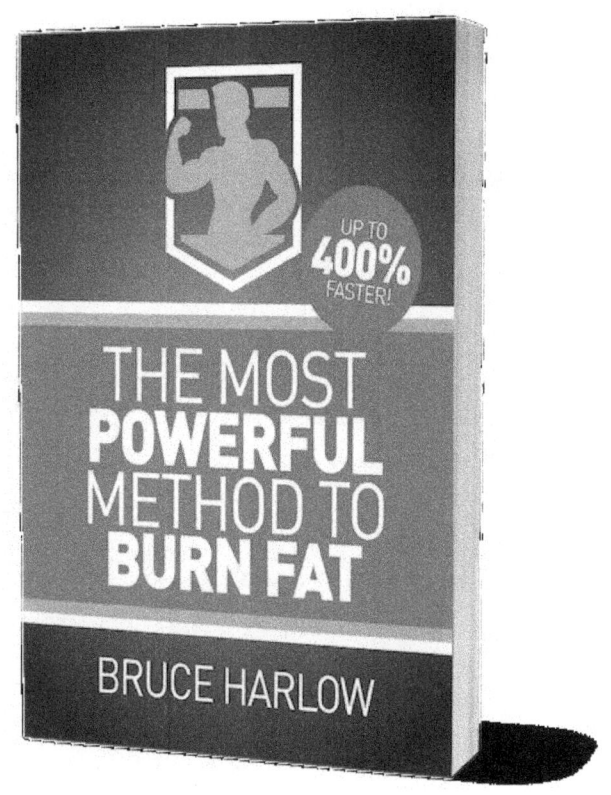

Get Your FREE Copy Here:
TopFitnessAdvice.com/Download

Conclusion

I hope that you have enjoyed these recipes and that you will have been inspired to try them out for yourself.

Once you understand something about how ketogenic recipes work, you can start to mix and match and experiment on your own.

With the great recipes in this book, you probably won't even feel like you are on diet. Losing weight could not be any easier.

Best of luck!

Don't forget to share your thoughts on this book by leaving a review on Amazon.com. It takes just a few seconds.

Enjoying this book?

Check out our other best sellers!

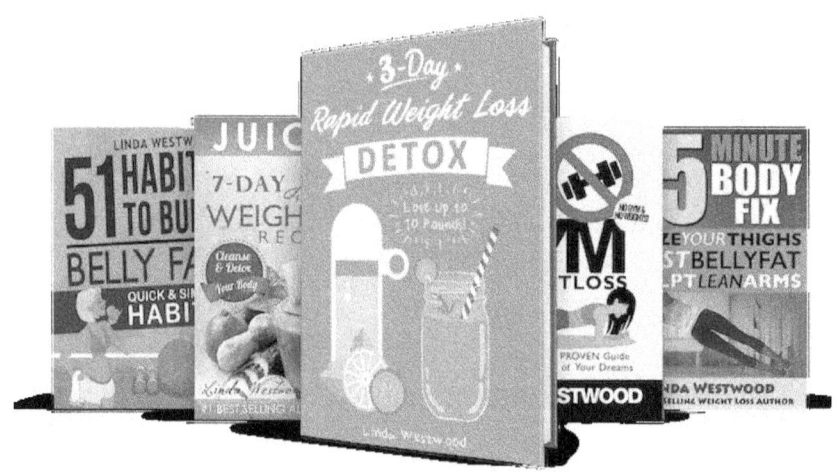

Get your next book on sale here:

TopFitnessAdvice.com/go/books

Final Words

I would like to thank you for purchasing my book and I hope I have been able to help you and educate you on something new.

If you have enjoyed this book and would like to share your positive thoughts, could you please take 30 seconds of your time to go back and give me a review on my Amazon book page.

I greatly appreciate seeing these reviews because it helps me share my hard work.

You can leave me a review on Amazon.com.

Again, thank you and I wish you all the best!

www.ingramcontent.com/pod-product-compliance
Lightning Source LLC
Chambersburg PA
CBHW031156020426
42333CB00013B/695